YOGA
FOR PREGNANCY

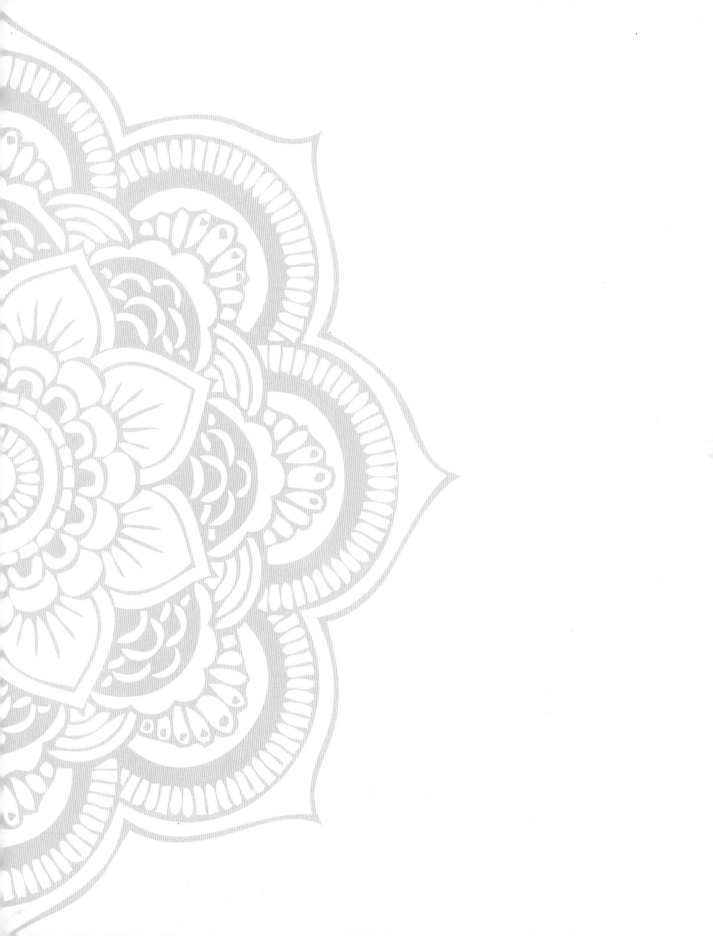

YOGA
FOR PREGNANCY

*Poses, Meditations, and Inspiration
for Expectant and New Mothers*

Leslie Lekos and Megan Westgate

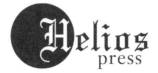

Helios
press

Copyright © 2014 by Leslie Lekos and Megan Westgate
Photographs copyright © 2014 by Jules Frazier

Helios Press books may be purchased in bulk at special discounts for sales promotion, corporate gifts, fund-raising, or educational purposes. Special editions can also be created to specifications. For details, contact the Special Sales Department, Helios Press, 307 West 36th Street, 11th Floor, New York, NY 10018 or info@skyhorsepublishing.com.

Helios Press is an imprint of Skyhorse Publishing. Skyhorse® and Skyhorse Publishing® are registered trademarks of Skyhorse Publishing, Inc.®, a Delaware corporation.

Visit our website at www.skyhorsepublishing.com.

10 9 8 7 6 5 4 3 2 1

Library of Congress Cataloging-in-Publication Data is available on file.

Cover photo by Jules Frazier

Print ISBN: 978-1-62914-362-0
Ebook ISBN: 978-1-63220-199-7

Printed in China

Contents

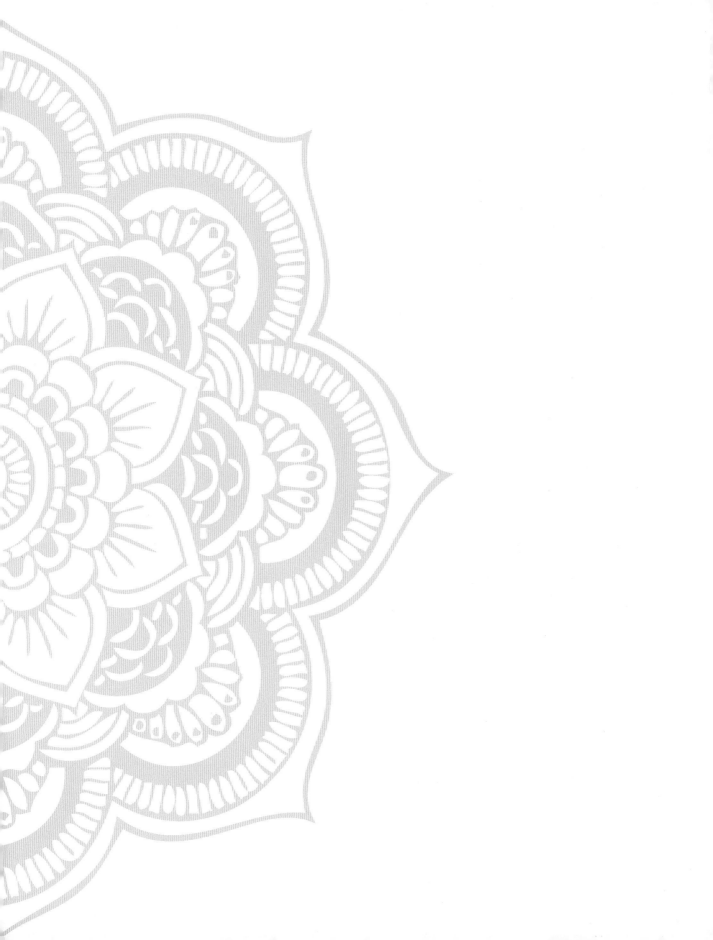

Introduction

Growing a baby is an honor and a responsibility unlike any other. A woman's practices during pregnancy lay the foundation for her birth experience and her child's constitution and lifelong development. Yoga is an amazing gift for both you and your baby as you begin this journey together.

This book was conceived when Megan was pregnant with her first child and a student in Leslie's prenatal yoga class. Both of us have been practicing yoga for fifteen years, and with Megan's passion for yoga philosophy and writing and Leslie's experience as a yoga teacher, childbirth educator, herbalist, and doula, we felt we could offer something valuable and unique to support pregnant women.

A primary inspiration is our mutual passion for alignment-based yoga. The first section of the book includes sixty-one poses (*asanas*) that are beneficial to practice while pregnant, and which will help you prepare for labor. Each one includes photographs as well as detailed instructions for how to practice the pose. Our guidance is focused on how each pose should *feel*, not just how it should look. Having appropriate engagement in the poses is especially important during pregnancy, when your body is producing extra relaxin hormone and your joints are looser.

The next section of the book is organized around the seven chakras, or energy centers, of the body. The practices for bringing balance to the chakras include asana sequences as well as mantras, visualizations, Kundalini meditations, and tea recipes inspired by Leslie's work as an herbalist.

In the third section, we offer a variety of poses to use during labor. Most of these are not traditional yoga poses; they are postures that Leslie has learned through her extensive experience as a doula.

Finally, we include practices for postpartum. Once you have your healthcare provider's approval to resume normal physical activity, the poses in this last section of the book can help you regain muscle tone and energy, and can support you in connecting with yourself and your baby.

We have created this book as a love-filled offering to every woman who is inspired to nourish herself and her baby with the myriad benefits of yoga. We wish you good health and many blessings on your amazing journey!

Namaste,

Leslie Lekos & Megan Westgate

July 2014

A Note to Practitioners

It is essential to listen deeply to your body throughout pregnancy and postpartum. A dedicated yoga practice is a wonderful tool for cultivating the kind of careful attention and listening that can help you stay safe and healthy throughout your pregnancy.

You should not feel pain in any of these yoga poses. The "Engaging actions" and "Details to be mindful of" given for the poses are designed to keep your practice safe and comfortable. If you experience persistent pain in a given pose, please discontinue practicing it and focus on the poses that feel helpful and nourishing to you.

In the first trimester, be extra gentle with yourself, particularly with back-bending actions. Deep back bends thin the belly and the uterine lining, which is not appropriate during pregnancy (the back bends section of this book contains only poses with very gentle back-bending action, which can be practiced safely).

If you had a confident and comfortable inversion practice prior to becoming pregnant, you may continue the poses presented in this book—with your health care provider's blessing—but be more cautious when kicking up. If these poses do not come easily to you, discontinue them during pregnancy.

Throughout pregnancy and particularly in the last trimester, as increased relaxin hormone levels loosen your muscles, tendons, and ligaments, be extra mindful not to overstretch in the poses. This also applies to the postpartum recovery period, when practice shifts to regaining strength and firmness throughout the body.

Always consult your health care provider before doing any physical program, including yoga, during the childbearing years.

Contraindicated Poses During Pregnancy

Avoid all twisting poses where the belly is compressed, for example:

- Marichyasana III (Seated Twist/Marichi's Pose)
- Parivritta Trikonasana (Revolved Triangle Pose)
- Parivritta Parsvakonasana (Revolved Side Angle Pose)
- Parivritta Ardha Chandrasana (Revolved Half Moon Pose)

Avoid all poses that compress the abdomen, for example:

- Urdhva Prasarita Padasana (Leg Lift)
- Paripurna Navasana (Boat Pose)
- Chaturanga Dandasana (Plank Pose/Four Limbed Staff Pose)
- Sit-ups

Avoid seated forward bends that put pressure on the belly, for example:

- Pascimottanasana (Seated Forward Fold)
- Janu Sirsasana (Head to Knee Forward Bend) (this can be safely modified, as shown on p. 85)
- Triang Mukaipada Pascimottanasana (Three Limbed One Foot Intense Stretch of the West) (this can be safely modified, as shown on p. 89)

Avoid back bends, except for the ones presented in this book. Most back bends have a thinning quality in the belly, for example:

- Urdhva Danurasana (Upward Bow Pose/ Wheel Pose)
- Ustrasana (Camel Pose)

Avoid poses that require you to lie on your belly, for example:

- Danurasana (Bow Pose)
- Salabasana (Locust Pose)

Avoid poses that require a rigorous kicking action, for example:

- Adho Mukha Vrksasana (Hand Stand)
- Pinchamayarasana (Elbow Balance)

Practitioners that have practiced Sirsasana and Sarvangasana proficiently and without difficulty prior to getting pregnant can continue them. When practiced with ease they are beneficial in supporting a healthy pregnancy. If these poses were not easy prior to pregnancy, discontinue them until after the postpartum period.

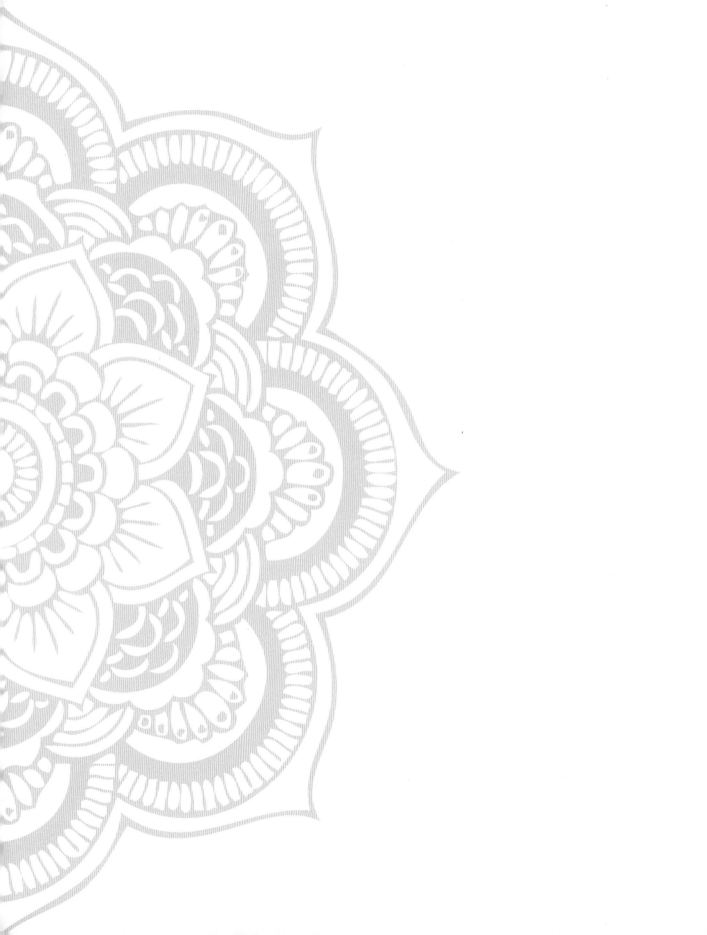

Visual Guide to Props

Using props in your practice can aid in better alignment, creating more space and freedom in the poses. This is especially helpful during pregnancy when props accommodate and support your changing body and make room for your growing baby. As props are mentioned throughout the book, reference this guide as needed.

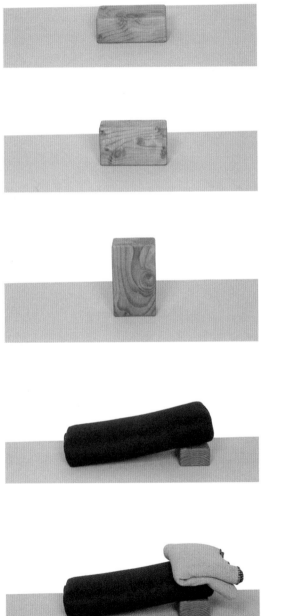

Low Block

Have the widest part of the block on the floor.

Medium Block

Turn the block up so it is lying on the long, thin side.

High Block

Turn the block up so the shortest, smallest edge of the block in touching the floor.

Supported Bolster

Place a low block toward the end of your sticky mat and prop up a bolster on top of the block. Be sure the block is right at the edge of the bolster so that your head will not droop down when you lie down on it.

Supported Bolster with Blanket

Follow the instructions for the supported bolster and place a basic fold blanket at the end of the bolster to be used as a pillow.

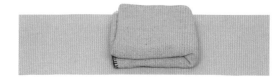

Basic Fold

Fold a blanket in half, joining the two longer edges together. Fold the blanket again, this time joining the two shorter ends. Do this a second time, joining the two shorter ends together. Now fold the blanket again, this time the opposite way, joining the outer edges of the blanket.

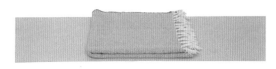

Open Fold

From Basic Fold, unfold the last fold of the blanket.

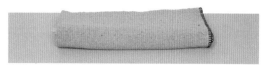

Narrow Fold

From Open Fold, fold the blanket on the length so it is long and narrow.

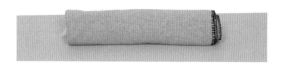

Roll

From Open Fold, roll the blanket from the longer side.

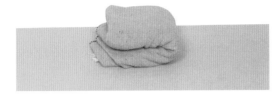

Side Lying Pillow Fold

From Basic Fold, fold the blanket in half again to make a square shape.

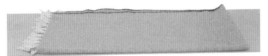

Open Open Fold

From Open Fold, open the blanket one more time.

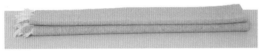

Narrow Trifold

From Open Open Fold, fold the blanket lengthwise in thirds. To do this, fold the blanket so a third is underneath and a third is on top. It folds together like an accordion.

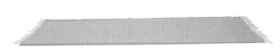

Half Fold

From Open Open Fold, open the blanket one more time.

Body Landmarks & Terms

Because of the emphasis on precise alignment and action, it is important to have a clear understanding of the terms used throughout the book to describe various parts of the body. Please use the chart below for reference.

NOTE

For ease of understanding, we have often opted to use common terms rather than anatomically correct ones (for example, "thigh bone" instead of "femur").

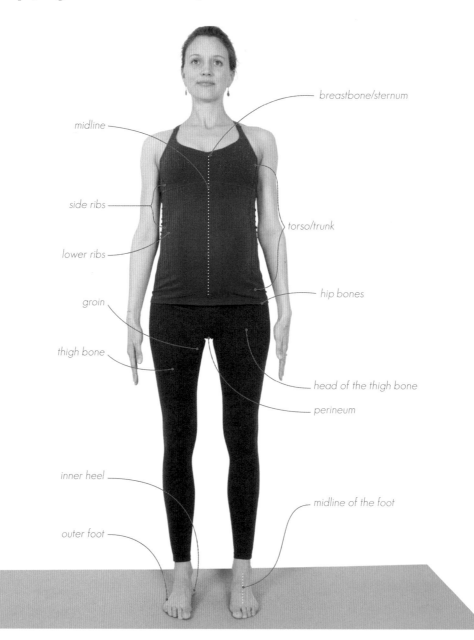

breastbone/sternum

midline

side ribs

torso/trunk

lower ribs

hip bones

groin

thigh bone

head of the thigh bone

perineum

inner heel

midline of the foot

outer foot

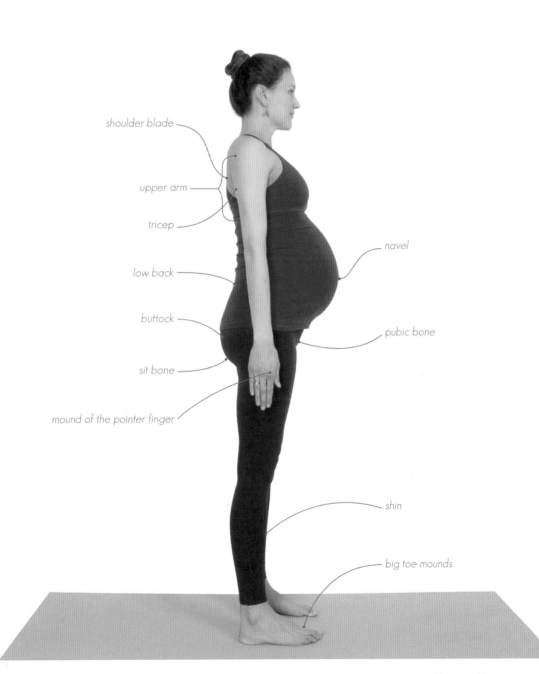

shoulder blade

upper arm

tricep

low back

buttock

sit bone

mound of the pointer finger

navel

pubic bone

shin

big toe mounds

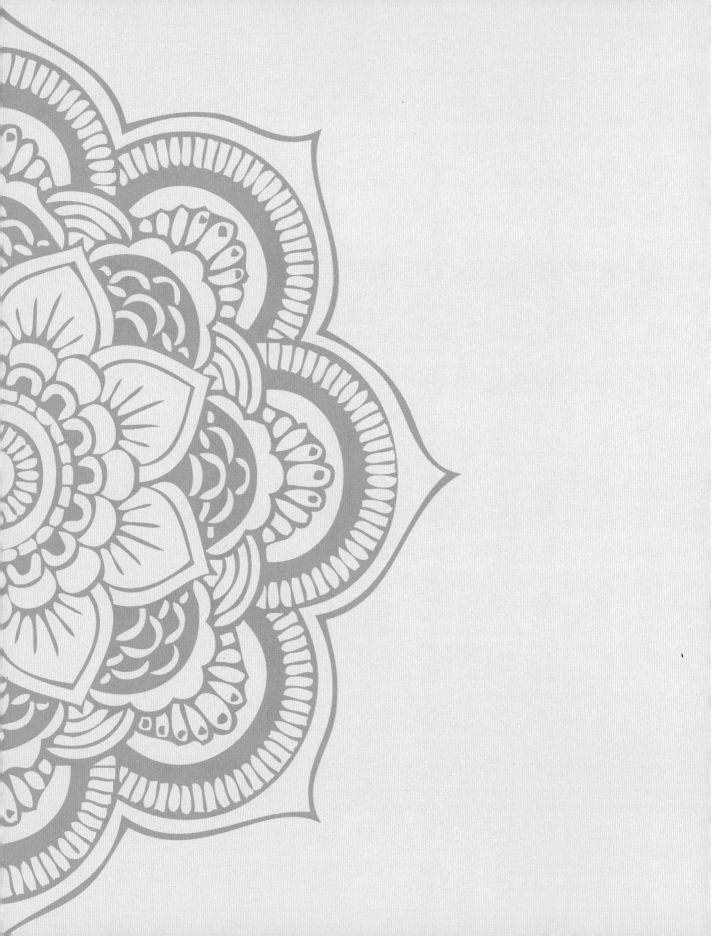

Poses and Practices for Pregnancy

Mindful asana practice brings a full spectrum of physical, mental, and emotional benefits during pregnancy. The instructions in this part of the book are based on three principles:

1. **Alignment.** The guidance for each "Getting into the pose" section informs you how to stack the bones for optimal anatomical alignment.

2. **Action.** Once your alignment is set, the "Engaging actions" section explains the movement and countermovement for each pose. You will notice that the emphasis is first on stability and then on stretching; these dual actions bring powerful, safe engagement in every pose.

3. **Breath.** Keeping attention on the breath is essential in order to fully experience the benefits of each pose. Breath instructions are included in the "Engaging actions," and each pose finishes with the important reminder to "soften your eyes, relax your face, and let the breath flow freely."

The pose begins after all the actions have been performed. See how much quietness you can find in each pose; experience the pose fully and discover what it has to offer you.

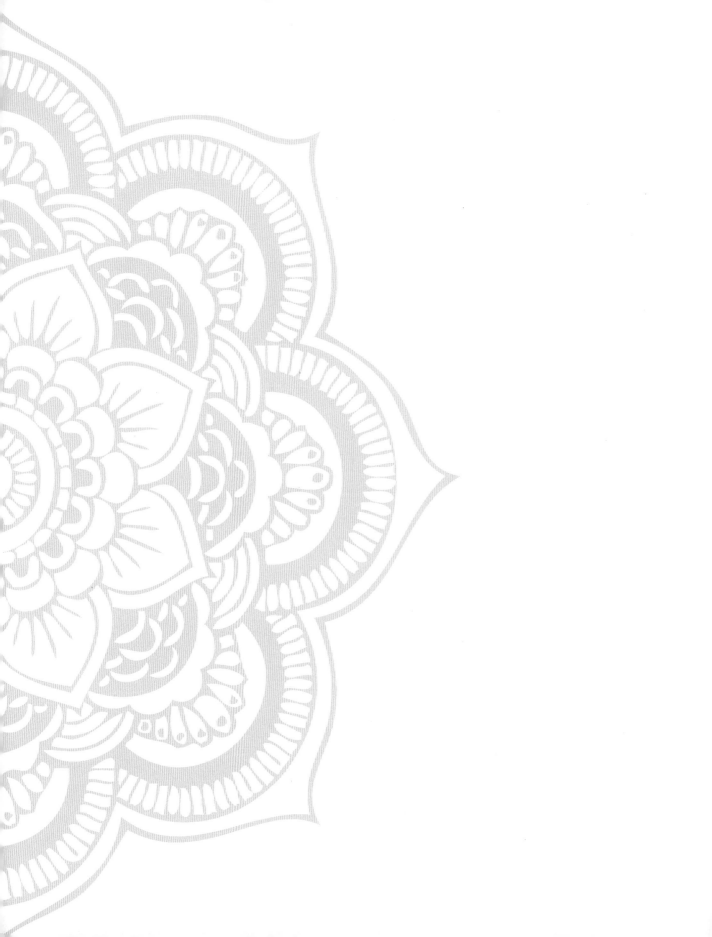

STANDING POSES

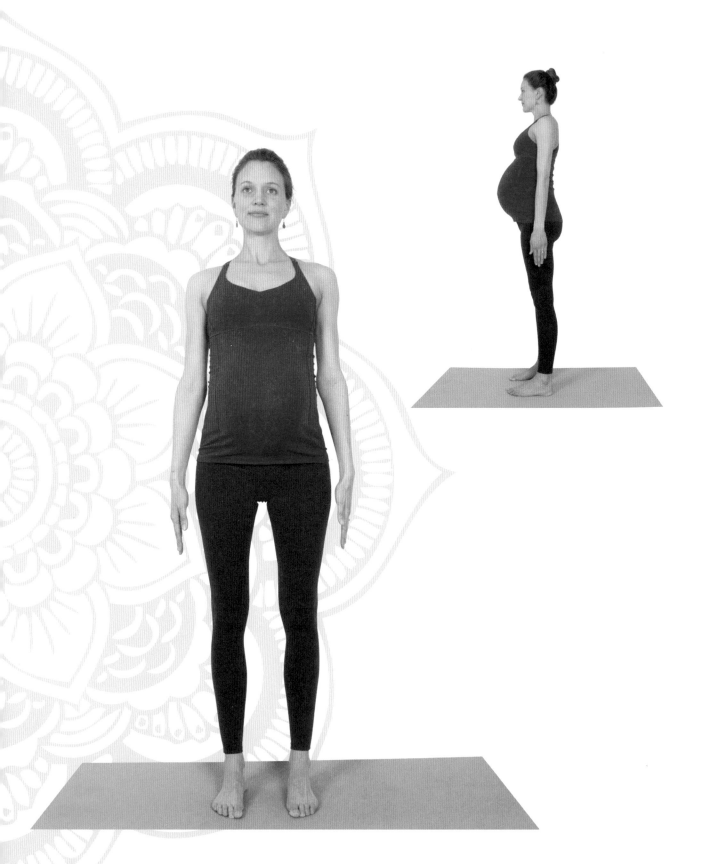

Tadasana
Mountain Pose

This is a foundational pose. Although it appears simple, the actions in Tadasana help inform proper engagement and alignment in all the other poses.

GETTING INTO THE POSE

1. Stand with your feet hip width apart.
2. The outer edges of your feet should be parallel and the midline of the feet pointing forward.

ENGAGING ACTIONS

1. Balance your weight equally between the feet and spread the toes.
2. Draw the tailbone in and the sitting bones down toward the backs of the knees.
3. Press the inner thighs back.
4. Draw the shoulders back and down.
5. Exhale; press your feet firmly down.
6. Inhale; lift the pubic bone toward the navel; lift your chest up; lift the side chest up.
7. Lift your kneecaps and firm the quadriceps.
8. Have your arms straight by your sides; extend the fingertips toward the floor.
9. Soften your eyes, relax your face, and let the breath flow freely.

Stay for 5–10 breaths.

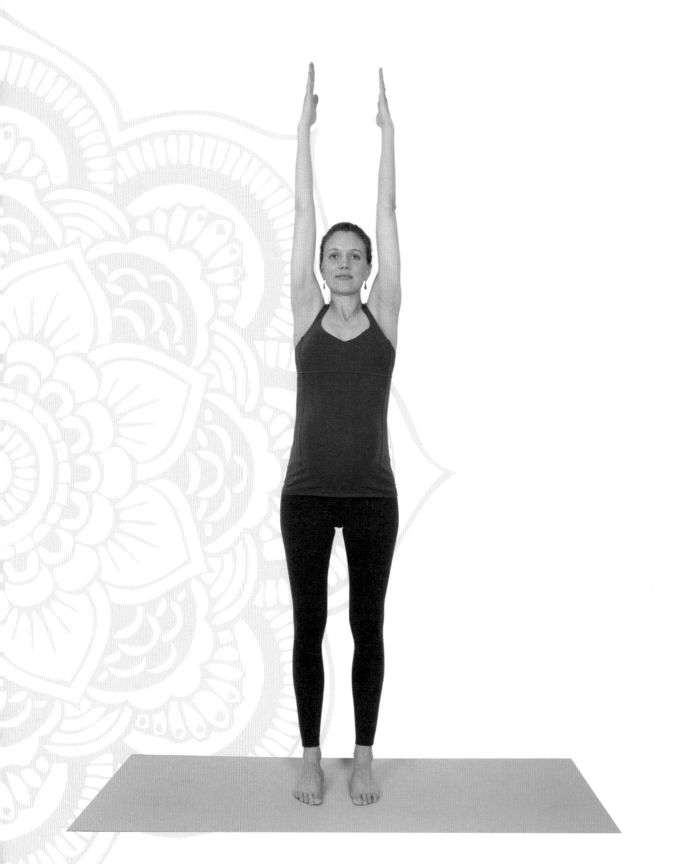

Urdhva Hastasana
Upward Hand Pose

This pose energizes the mind and body and teaches proper extension of the arms.

GETTING INTO THE POSE

1. Stand in Tadasana.
2. Extend your arms up over the head with the wrists shoulder width apart and palms facing each other; the arms should be parallel to each other and in line with the ears.

ENGAGING ACTIONS

1. Rotate the upper arms in.
2. Draw the inner shoulder blades down.
3. Draw the tailbone in and the sitting bones down toward the backs of the knees.
4. Exhale; press the feet firmly into the floor.
5. Inhale; lift and broaden the chest; lift the quadriceps up; lift the kneecaps up.
6. Extend strongly through the fingertips, straighten your arms up fully, and firm the muscles of the arms.
7. Soften your eyes, relax your face, and let the breath flow freely.

Stay for 5–10 breaths.

COMING OUT OF THE POSE

Release the arms down by your sides and return to Tadasana.

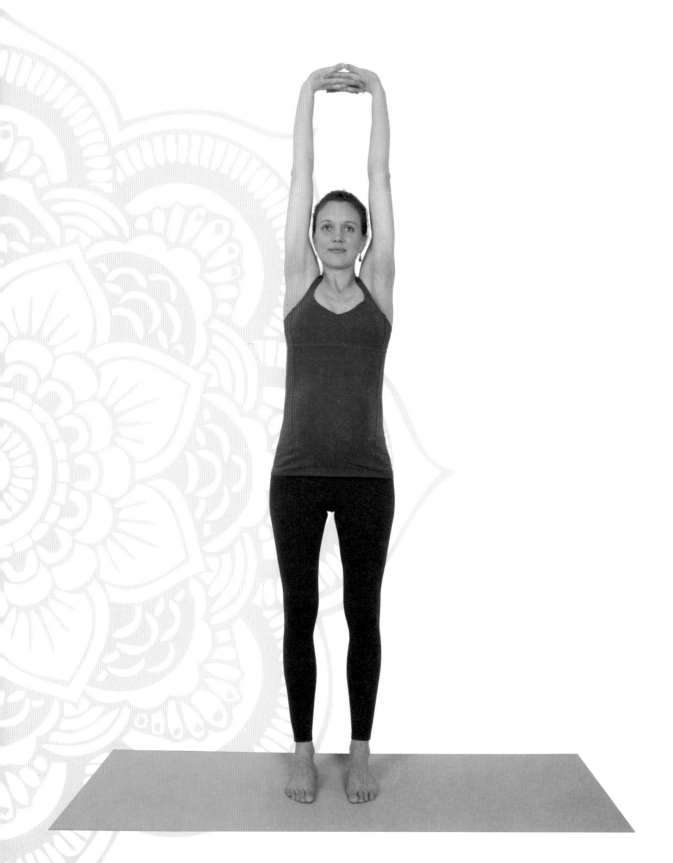

Urdhva Baddhanguliyasana

Upward Bound Hands Pose

This pose opens the chest, strengthens the arms, and is uplifting to the spirit.

Getting into the Pose

1. Stand in Tadasana.
2. Extend your arms out in front of you, parallel with the floor.
3. Interlace your hands all the way up to the webbing of your fingers and turn your palms away from you.
4. Lift your arms up over your head.
5. Extend the mound of the pointer fingers up and draw the little fingers back and down toward your head; the arms should be parallel to each other and in line with the ears.

Engaging Actions

1. Draw the tailbone in and the sitting bones down toward the backs of the knees.
2. Exhale; press the feet firmly down.
3. Inhale; lift and broaden the chest; lift the sides of your chest higher.
4. Extend your arms fully.
5. Soften your eyes, relax your face, and let the breath flow freely.

Details to Be Mindful Of

To keep from overarching the back, draw the front ribs into the back body while still maintaining the lift of the chest.

Stay for 5–10 breaths.

Coming Out of the Pose

Release the arms down by your sides and return to Tadasana.

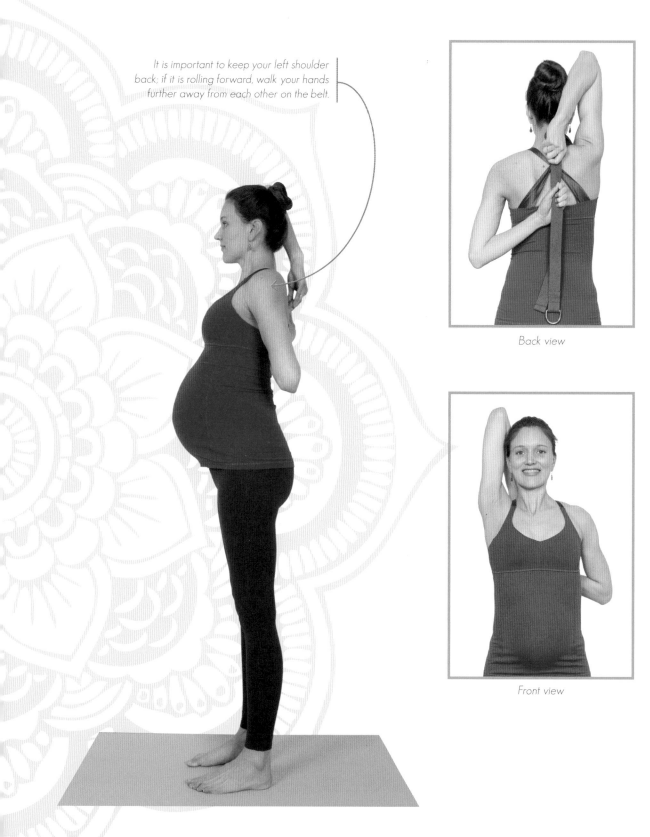

It is important to keep your left shoulder back; if it is rolling forward, walk your hands further away from each other on the belt.

Back view

Front view

Gomukasana in Tadasana

Cow Face in Mountain Pose

This pose opens the shoulders and can be helpful in resolving neck issues.

NOTE

If you have shoulder issues and feel strain in this posture, back off or discontinue the pose altogether.

GETTING INTO THE POSE

1. Stand in Tadasana.
2. Place a belt over the right shoulder.
3. Extend the right arm up to the ceiling and turn the palm back.
4. Bend the elbow and take hold of the belt with your right hand behind your back.
5. Point your right elbow straight to the ceiling and rotate the tricep muscle in toward your midline.
6. Maintain those movements in the right arm and take the left arm out to the left side, parallel with the floor.
7. Turn the left thumb down and palm back.
8. Bend the elbow and take hold of the belt behind the back.
9. Walk your hands as close together as you can; if you can grip the hands together then do so.

ENGAGING ACTIONS

1. Draw the left shoulder back and take the left shoulder blade into the body to open the chest further.
2. Draw the tailbone in and the sitting bones down toward the backs of the knees.
3. Exhale; press the feet firmly down.
4. Inhale; lift and broaden the chest up; lift the sides of your chest higher up.
5. Soften your eyes, relax your face, and let the breath flow freely.

DETAILS TO BE MINDFUL OF

- To keep from overarching the back, draw the front ribs into the back body while still maintaining the lift of the chest.
- Keep the head in line with the spine.

Stay for 5–10 breaths.

COMING OUT OF THE POSE

1. Release the grip and extend the arms wide.
2. Return to Tadasana.

Repeat on the other side.

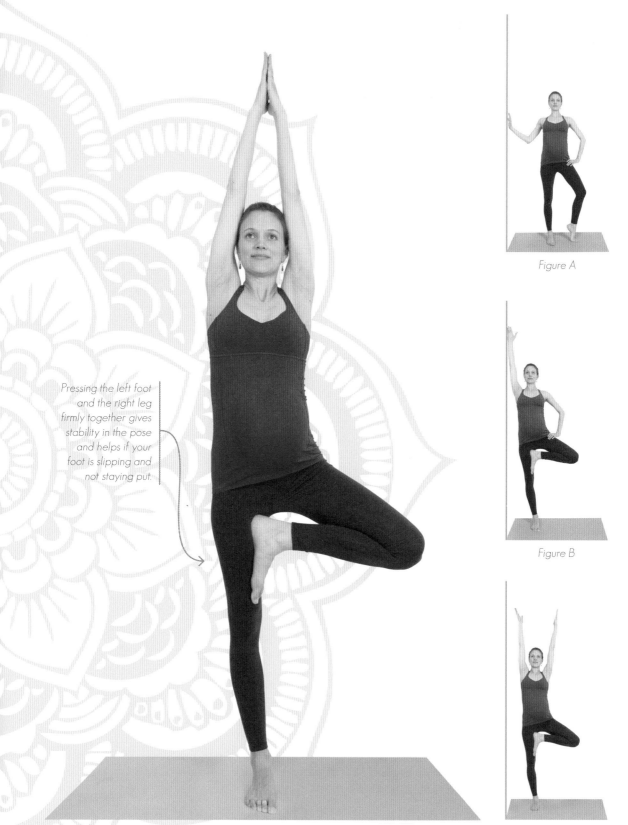

Pressing the left foot and the right leg firmly together gives stability in the pose and helps if your foot is slipping and not staying put.

Figure A

Figure B

Figure C

Vrksasana
Tree Pose

This pose teaches balance, which is ever changing during pregnancy as the baby shifts and grows. Vrksasana brings focus to the mind, is strengthening to the arms and legs, and opens the hips.

Getting into the pose

1. Stand in Tadasana with the wall on your right side.
2. Place your left hand on your hip and your right fingertips on the wall, right elbow slightly bent.
3. Bend your left knee and rotate your left thigh out to the side *(Figure A)*.
4. Take hold of your left ankle and place your left foot as high up as you can on your right thigh with your left toes pointing straight down toward the floor.
5. Keep your hip bones facing evenly forward.
6. Walk your right hand up the wall *(Figure B)*.
7. Raise your left arm up and reach strongly through your fingertips.
8. Turn the right palm so the back of the hand is against the wall.
9. If you're working on balancing, stay in this variation.
10. If you have the balance, take your right hand away from the wall. Have your arms in line with your ears and palms facing each other shoulder width apart *(Figure C)* or take the palms together.
11. Roll the upper arms in strongly and straighten the arms fully.

Engaging actions

1. Draw the tailbone in.
2. Exhale; press your right foot firmly into the floor, especially the right inner heel.
3. Inhale; lift the chest up, lift the sides of your chest higher, and extend fully through the fingertips.
4. Lift the right kneecap and firm the leg.
5. Soften your eyes, relax your face, and let the breath flow freely.

Stay for 5–10 breaths.

Note

If you can't have your foot higher than your knee, place your foot below your knee to avoid having the foot pressing on the knee joint.

Coming out of the pose

Maintaining steadiness and keeping the chest lifted, release your left foot and return to Tadasana.

Repeat on the other side.

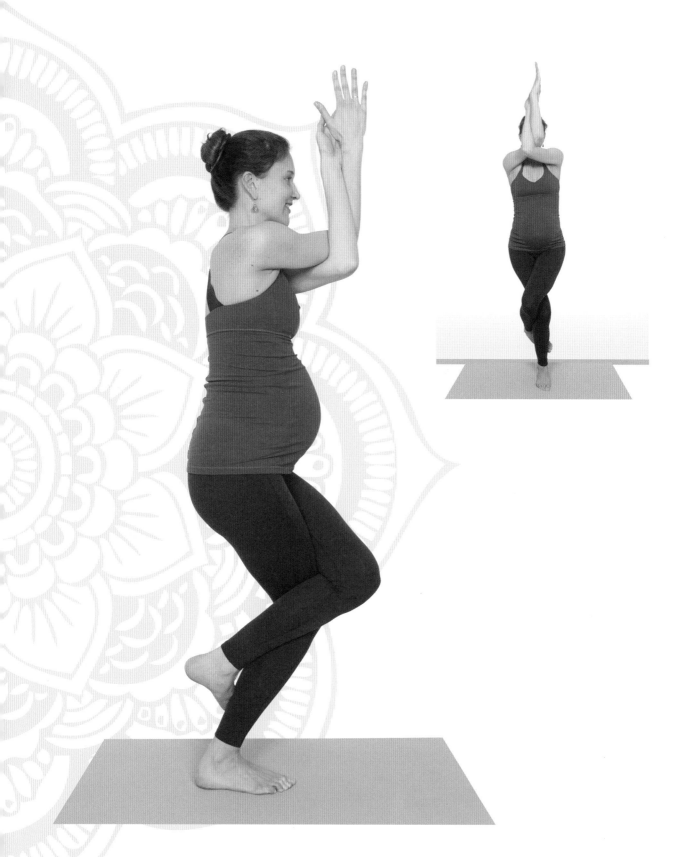

Garudasana

Eagle Pose

This pose releases upper back tension. It also teaches balance and focus.

NOTE

This pose should not be practiced in the third trimester of pregnancy, as the thighs pressing together make less space for baby. During pregnancy, it is recommended that you practice this pose with your back against the wall for stability and to prevent abdominal strain; be sure that the buttock, back, and head are all touching the wall.

GETTING INTO THE POSE

1. Stand in Tadasana with your back and head against the wall.
2. Bend your knees slightly.
3. Raise your left leg and take the left thigh over the right thigh.
4. If you can, hook the left foot behind the right calf as shown; if this is not possible, instead press the left little toe to the outer right calf.
5. Extend your arms out in front of you, parallel with the floor.
6. Cross your right arm over your left arm, just above the elbow.
7. Bend both elbows and point your fingers up toward the ceiling.
8. Join your palms together; if this is not possible, hook the left pinky finger with the right thumb.

ENGAGING ACTIONS

1. Draw the heads of your shoulders back to the wall and down, away from your ears.
2. Extend the elbows away from the trunk and lift the fingers up so the upper arms are parallel with the floor.
3. Draw the tailbone in and the sitting bones down toward the backs of the knees.
4. Exhale; press the right foot down, especially the right inner heel.
5. Inhale; lift and broaden the chest; lift the sides of your chest.
6. Soften your eyes, relax your face, and let the breath flow freely.

Stay for 3–4 breaths.

COMING OUT OF THE POSE

1. Release the arms.
2. Unwind your legs and return to Tadasana.

Repeat on the other side.

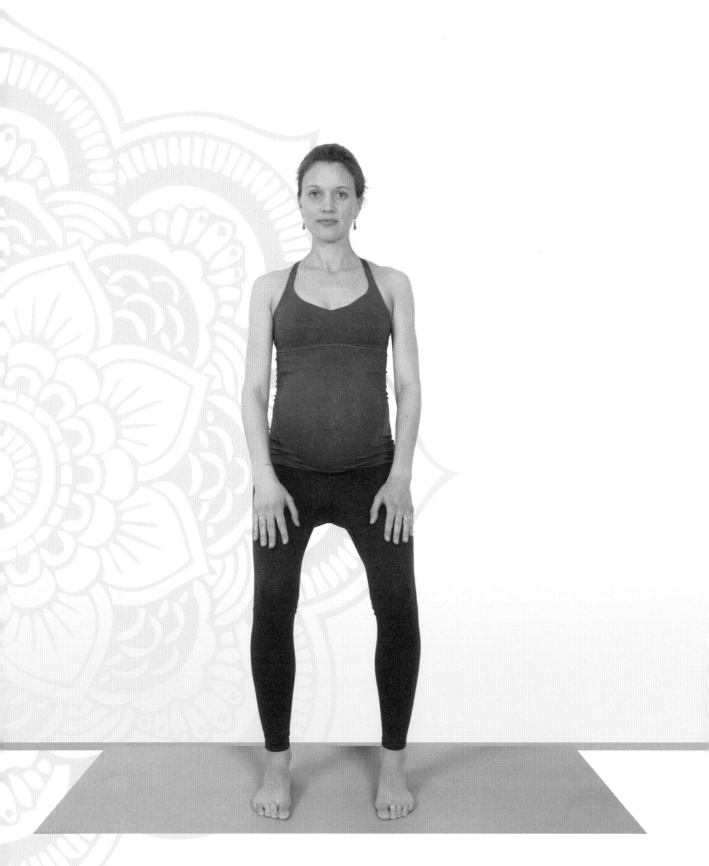

Utkatasana
Fierce Pose/Chair Pose

This is an excellent pose to release tension in the low back. It is also very strengthening for the legs.

NOTE

This dynamic adaptation of Utkatasana uses movement to release the low back and is a variation that is safe during pregnancy. The wall provides stability and support during pregnancy; be sure that the buttock, shoulders, and head are all touching the wall.

GETTING INTO THE POSE

1. Stand in Tadasana, about six inches away from the wall.
2. Be sure that the outer feet are parallel with each other and the midline of the feet are pointing straight forward.
3. Bend the knees and rest the back and head against the wall.
4. Rest the hands on the thighs.

ENGAGING ACTIONS

1. Exhale; press the heels firmly down.
2. Inhale; lift and broaden the chest.
3. Exhale; lift the pubic bone toward the navel, drawing the belly into the spine and pressing the low back to the wall.
4. With your next inhalation, tilt your pelvis forward so that there is space between the low back and the wall.

DETAILS TO BE MINDFUL OF

- Pay attention to the two sides of the spine as you do the pelvic rocking motion; notice if both sides press equally to the wall as you move.
- Move slowly, vertebrae by vertebrae, during each inhalation and exhalation to deepen your awareness of your low back.

Continue this rhythm for 8–10 breaths.

NOTE

This is the same action as in Cat/Cow (p. 119).

COMING OUT OF THE POSE

Straighten the legs and return to Tadasana.

VARIATIONS

To intensify the pose, extend the arms up to the ceiling as in Urdhva Hastasana (p. 17) and/or bend the knees more deeply.

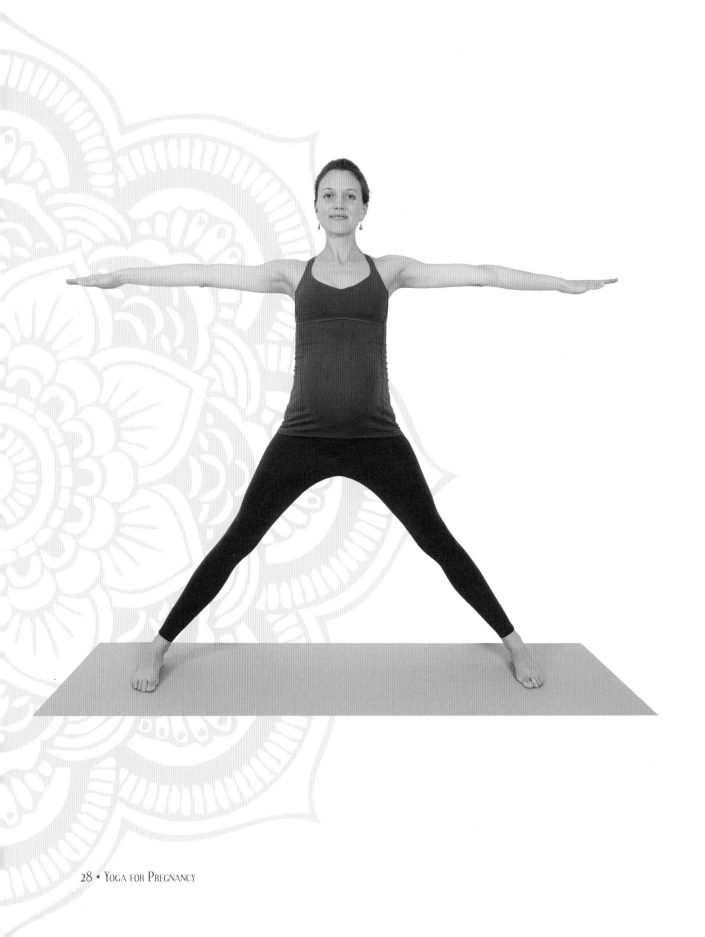

Utthita Hasta Padasana
Extended Hand Foot Pose

This pose and Parsva Hasta Padasana (next page) are used in setting up many of the other standing poses. A solid foundation in Utthita Hasta Padasana will bring stability to the other poses you transition into from here.

Getting into the Pose

1. Stand in Tadasana in the middle of your sticky mat.
2. Step your feet 3½ to 4 feet apart.
3. Turn your toes in slightly so the outer edges of your feet are parallel.
4. Extend your arms wide so the fingertips, wrists, and shoulders are in line; your arms are parallel to the floor.

Engaging actions

1. Exhale; press your outer feet down.
2. Inhale; lift and broaden your chest; lift your side ribs.
3. Lift your kneecaps, quadriceps, and inner thighs up.
4. Soften your eyes, relax your face, and let the breath flow freely.

Details to be mindful of

Keep the head in line with the spine.

Stay for 5 breaths.

Coming out of the Pose

Return to Tadasana.

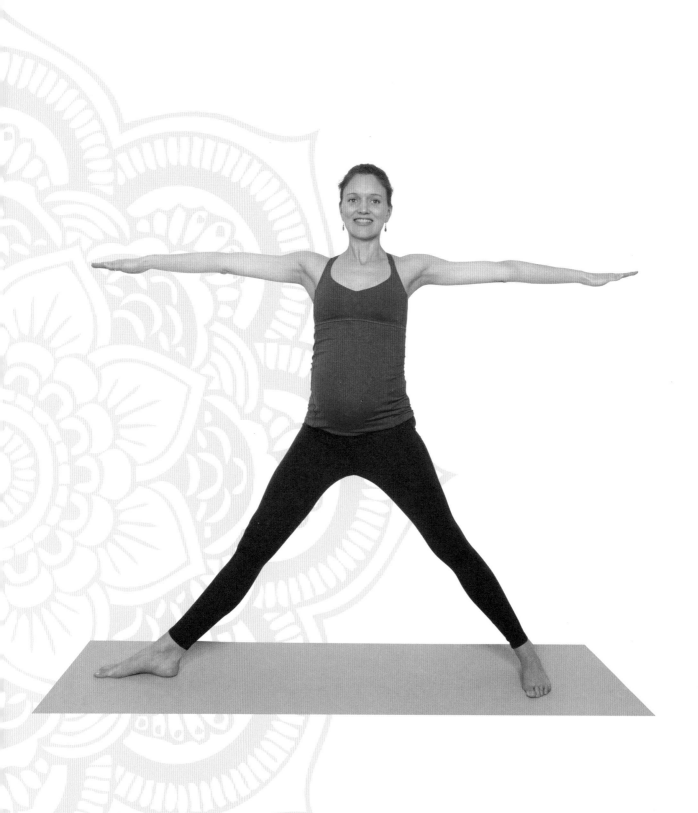

Parsva Hasta Padasana
Side Hand Foot Pose

This pose and Utthita Hasta Padasana (previous page) are used in setting up many of the other standing poses. A solid foundation in Parsva Hasta Padasana will bring stability to the other poses you transition into from here.

Getting into the pose

1. Stand in Tadasana in the middle of your sticky mat.
2. Step into Utthita Hasta Padasana (previous page).
3. Turn your left foot in slightly.
4. Turn your right foot out 90 degrees.
5. Line up your right heel with your left arch.
6. Rotate your chest straight forward.

Engaging actions

1. Draw the tailbone in and the sitting bones down toward the backs of your knees.
2. Rotate the inner right thigh out to line up the center of your knee with the center of your foot.
3. Exhale; press your feet firmly down, especially your left outer foot, and lift the kneecaps.
4. Inhale; lift and broaden your chest; lift your side ribs up.
5. Soften your eyes, relax your face, and let the breath flow freely.

Stay for 5 breaths.

Coming out of the pose

1. Rotate your feet back to Utthita Hasta Padasana.
2. Return to Tadasana.

Repeat on the other side.

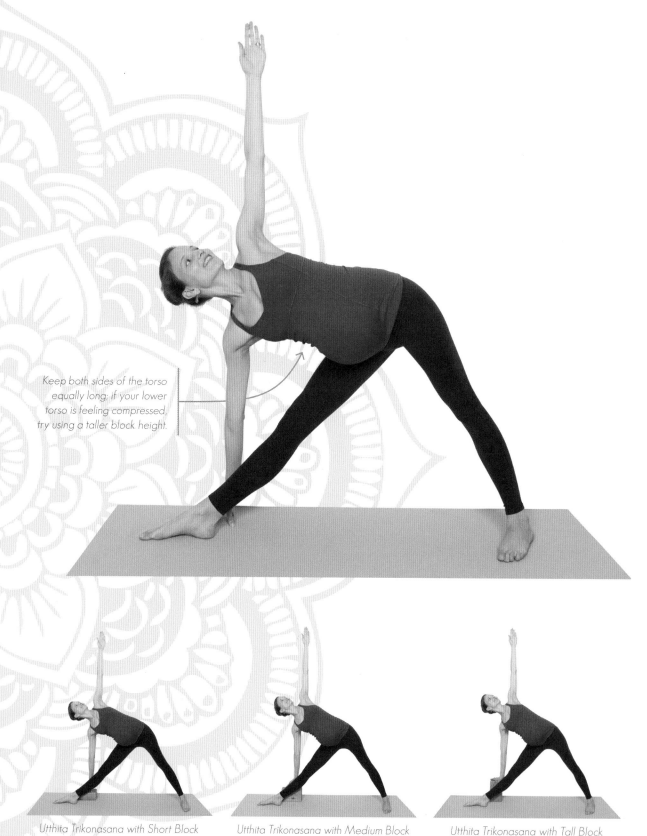

Keep both sides of the torso equally long; if your lower torso is feeling compressed, try using a taller block height.

Utthita Trikonasana with Short Block   Utthita Trikonasana with Medium Block   Utthita Trikonasana with Tall Block

Utthita Trikonasana

Extended Triangle Pose

This pose strengthens the legs, arms, and spine. It helps generate stability and stamina.

Getting into the pose

1. Set up 2 blocks at the back of your mat on the short height (see p. 5), about 3½ to 4 feet apart.
2. Stand in Tadasana in the middle of your sticky mat.
3. Step into Utthita Hasta Padasana (p. 29).
4. Rotate into Parsva Hasta Padasana (previous page).
5. Take the hands to the hips.
6. Line up the right heel with the arch of the left foot.
7. Rotate the inner right thigh out to line up the center of your knee with the center of your foot.
8. Rotate the chest straight forward.
9. Press your outer left foot firmly to the floor.
10. Bend from your right hip crease and place your right hand on the block.
11. Move the block so that the right wrist is directly under the right shoulder.
12. Have the left hand on your left hip and rotate the left elbow and shoulder back.
13. Take the right chest and right buttock forward.
14. Extend your left arm up; keep pressing the right hand down and extend strongly up through the left fingertips to broaden the chest.

Engaging actions

1. Exhale; press your feet firmly down, especially the outer left foot.
2. Inhale; draw the sternum bone away from the navel, draw the kneecaps up, and firm the quadriceps muscles.
3. Rotate your belly and chest up to the ceiling and look up if that feels good, or you can keep your gaze focused straight ahead.
4. Soften your eyes, relax your face, and let the breath flow freely.

Details to be mindful of

Keep both legs straight, with the leg muscles firm.

Stay for 5–10 breaths.

Coming out of the pose

1. Look straight forward, press the feet firmly down, and reach up with the left fingertips to lift yourself back to Parsva Hasta Padasana.
2. Rotate your feet back to Utthita Hasta Padasana.
3. Return to Tadasana.

Repeat on the left side.

During the first and second trimester, bend your knee as close to 90 degrees as possible, so that your front thigh is parallel to the floor. During the third trimester, protect your hypermobile joints by bending less or doing the chair variation.

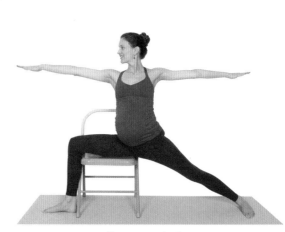

Variation: with chair

Virabhadrasana II
Warrior II Pose

Virabhadrasana II is uplifting and generates heat. It is strengthening for the legs, which in turn helps support the spine.

NOTE

For extra stability, you can practice this pose with your back heel against the wall. This is especially helpful if you are experiencing discomfort in your sacral iliac joint. If the strain persists, or in later stages of pregnancy when there is more relaxin in the body, back off or discontinue the pose altogether.

Discontinue this pose toward the end of pregnancy (after about 34 weeks) if baby is not head down.

GETTING INTO THE POSE

1. Stand in Tadasana in the middle of your sticky mat.
2. Step into Utthita Hasta Padasana (p. 29).
3. Rotate into Parsva Hasta Padasana (p. 31) on the right side.
4. Press firmly into the outer left foot and bend the right knee so that the center of the knee is in line with the center of the foot and the knee is in line with the ankle.
5. Keep the chest facing straight forward and extend through the arms and fingertips strongly to open the chest, wrists in line with the shoulders.

ENGAGING ACTIONS

1. Draw the tailbone in and the sitting bones down toward the backs of the knees.
2. Exhale; press the feet firmly down, especially the outer left foot.
3. Inhale; lift the chest up, lift the sides of your chest up higher and firm the left leg.
4. Keep the head in line with the spine and turn your head to look over the right fingertips.
5. Soften your eyes, relax your face, and let the breath flow freely.

DETAILS TO BE MINDFUL OF

- There is a tendency to lean the torso toward the bent leg; be sure to keep your spine perfectly vertical.
- Check to make sure the bent knee is in line with the ankle and the center of the knee is in line with the center of the foot.

Stay for 5–10 breaths.

COMING OUT OF THE POSE

1. Press your feet down and reach through the left fingertips to straighten your right leg and come up.
2. Rotate your feet back to Utthita Hasta Padasana.
3. Step your feet back together.
4. Return to Tadasana.

Repeat on the other side.

VARIATION: WITH CHAIR

You can also do this pose seated on a chair. This is a good way to practice at later stages of pregnancy.

In this variation be mindful to really press into the back outer foot and straighten that leg fully. Also, check to make sure the bent knee is in line with the center of the foot and is also in line with the ankle.

Keep both sides of the torso equally long; if your lower torso is feeling compressed, try using a taller block height.

Press the outer right knee into the right arm for stability.

During the first and second trimester, bend your knee as close to 90 degrees as possible, so that your bent thigh is parallel to the floor; during the third trimester, protect your hypermobile joints by bending less.

Utthita Parsvakonasana
Extended Side Angle Pose

This pose creates openness and space in the ribs, which can bring ease to the breath, make more room for baby, and release tension in the upper body. It also opens the hips, strengthens the legs, and supports healthy digestion.

NOTE

In later stages of pregnancy when there is more relaxin in the body, back off or discontinue the pose altogether. Also discontinue this pose toward the end of pregnancy (after about 34 weeks) if baby is not head down.

GETTING INTO THE POSE

1. Set up 2 blocks on the low height at the back of your mat, about 3½ to 4 feet apart.
2. Stand in Tadasana in the middle of your sticky mat.
3. Step into Utthita Hasta Padasana (p. 29).
4. Rotate your feet into Parsva Hasta Padasana (p. 31).
5. Press firmly into the outer left foot and bend the right knee so that the center of the knee is in line with the center of the foot and the knee is in line with the ankle.
6. Bend from your hip to place the right hand on the block.
7. Move the block so the wrist and shoulder are in line.
8. Press your right outer knee into your arm, keeping the knee in line with the midline of your foot.
9. Place the left hand on the left hip; rotate the left elbow and shoulder back and the right chest and right buttock forward so the whole belly and chest rotate toward the ceiling.
10. Extend your left arm out and reach your fingertips back toward your left foot side, wrist in line with the shoulder and arm parallel with the floor.
11. Turn the left palm up and reach the arm over the head, feeling one line of energy from your outer left foot through your left fingertips.

ENGAGING ACTIONS

1. Draw the tailbone in.
2. Draw the shoulders away from the ears.
3. Exhale; press the feet firmly down, especially the left outer foot.
4. Inhale; draw the sternum bone away from the navel; firm your left thigh.
5. Rotate your belly and chest up to the ceiling even more and look up to the inside of your arm if that feels good, or you can keep your gaze focused straight ahead.
6. Soften your eyes, relax your face and let the breath flow freely.

DETAILS TO BE MINDFUL OF

To keep from overarching your back, draw your lower ribs in, move the right sitting bone forward, and press the inner left thigh back.

Stay for 5–10 breaths.

COMING OUT OF THE POSE

1. Rotate your gaze back so you are looking forward.
2. Lower your left arm back to shoulder height.
3. Press your feet firmly down, especially the outer left foot, and reach through the left fingertips to lift up out of the pose.
4. Straighten your right leg into Utthita Parsva Hastasana (p. 31).
5. Rotate your feet and chest back to Utthita Hasta Padasana (p. 29).
6. Return to Tadasana.

Repeat on the other side.

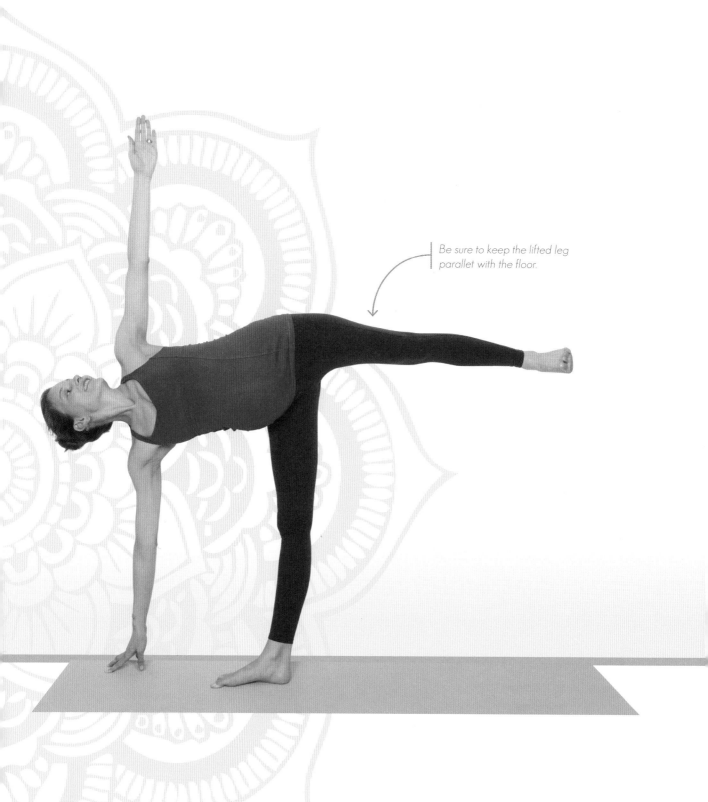

Be sure to keep the lifted leg parallel with the floor.

Ardha Chandrasana
Half Moon Pose

Ardha Chandrasana is an uplifting balancing pose that can relieve nausea and fatigue. It brings expansion and lightness to the body, making space for baby.

NOTE

During pregnancy, it is recommended that you practice this pose against the wall for stability and support; be sure that the buttock is touching the wall.

GETTING INTO THE POSE

1. Set up 2 blocks on the tall height (see p. 5) against the wall at the back of your mat, about 3½ to 4 feet apart.
2. Stand with your heels a few inches away from the wall in Utthita Hasta Padasana (p. 29); your buttock should be lightly touching the wall or very close to it.
3. Come into Utthita Trikonasana (p. 33), on the right side, then bend your right knee.
4. Take the block about 12 inches beyond your right foot and against the wall.
5. Place the left hand on the left hip; rotate the left elbow and shoulder back to the wall and the right chest and right buttock forward so the whole belly and chest rotate toward the ceiling.
6. Keeping the rotation, lift the left leg up so that it is parallel with the floor and straighten your right leg.
7. Extend and reach the left fingertips toward the ceiling; both the wrists should be in line with the shoulders.

ENGAGING ACTIONS

1. Exhale; press strongly through the inner heels and big toe mounds.
2. Inhale; take the sternum bone away from the navel and extend strongly through the left fingertips.
3. Straighten both legs fully and firm the inner knees.
4. Rotate your belly and chest up to the ceiling even more.
5. Soften your eyes, relax your face, and let the breath flow freely.

DETAILS TO BE MINDFUL OF

- Find the right block height for you—your chest should not be much lower than your hips during pregnancy; if it is, then remedy this by bringing your block to a taller height.
- Your right hip should be directly over your right ankle.
- Make sure that the center of your right foot faces straight forward.

Stay for 3–4 breaths.

COMING OUT OF THE POSE

1. Bend the right knee; place your left foot on the floor.
2. Return to Utthita Trikonasana (p. 33).
3. Look straight forward, press the feet firmly down and reach through the left fingertips to bring yourself back up to Parsva Hasta Padasana (p. 31).
4. Come into Uttitha Hasta Padasana (p. 29).

Repeat on the other side.

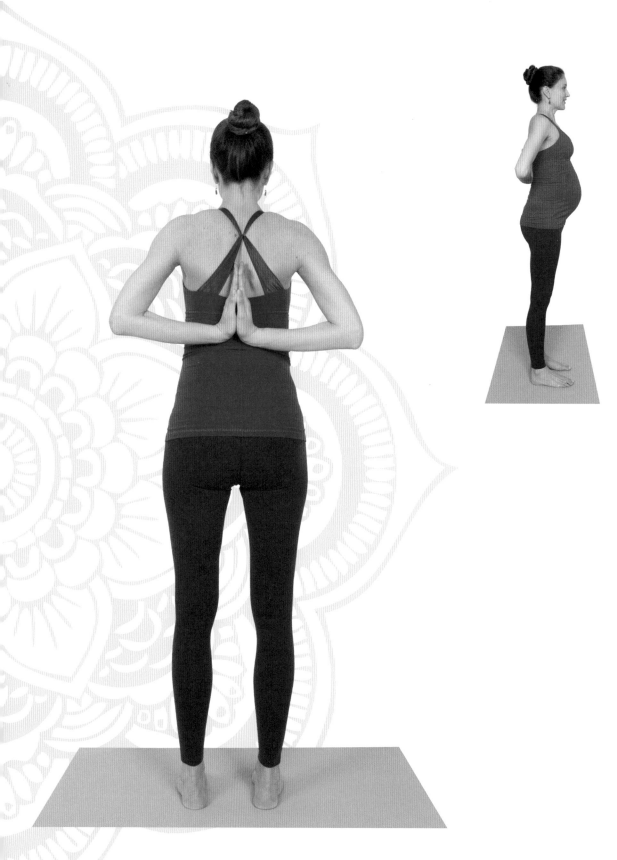

Paschima Namaskarasana in Tadasana

Reverse Prayer Pose in Mountain Pose

This pose opens the shoulders and chest and brings freedom to the neck. The hand position and arm actions are the same as for the classic version of Parsvottanasana (next page).

GETTING INTO THE POSE

1. Stand in Tadasana.
2. Extend your arms wide out to the sides, wrists in line with the shoulders, arms parallel to the floor.
3. Take your palms together behind your back, fingers pointing toward floor.
4. Turn your palms up so the fingers point toward the ceiling; work your hands as high up the back as you can.
5. Press the hands together strongly, sealing the palms together.

ENGAGING ACTIONS

1. Draw the outer shoulders back and the inner shoulder blades in.
2. Draw the sitting bones down and the tailbone in.
3. Exhale; spread the toes and press the feet firmly down.
4. Inhale; lift and broaden the chest; lift the kneecaps up; firm your legs.
5. Soften your eyes, relax your face, and let the breath flow freely.

DETAILS TO BE MINDFUL OF

- To keep from overarching the back, draw the front ribs into the back body and press the inner thighs back.
- If you cannot take your hands into this position, clasp your elbows or wrists behind your back with your hands instead.

Stay for 5 breaths.

COMING OUT OF THE POSE

Extend the arms wide, then release them down to your sides and return to Tadasana.

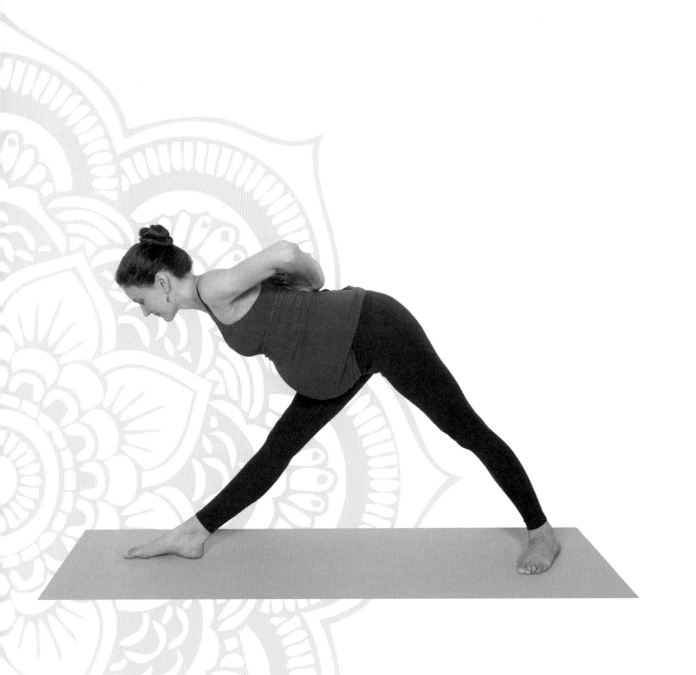

Parsvottanasana

Intense Side Stretch Pose

Parsvottanasana stretches the legs and opens the shoulders, sides, and upper back. Practicing this pose is believed to make delivery easier.

NOTE

Be careful to avoid compressing the belly against the thigh. In later stages of pregnancy you will not be able to go as far forward.

GETTING INTO THE POSE

1. Stand in Tadasana.
2. Bring your hands into Paschima Namaskara in Tadasana (previous page); if you cannot have the hands in this position, clasp your elbows or wrists behind your back instead.
3. Step into Utthita Hasta Padasana (p. 29).
4. Turn your left foot in 80 degrees and your right foot out 90 degrees.
5. Line up your right heel with your left arch; if you're having trouble balancing you can widen your stance, so your heels are in line with each other.
6. Draw your right hip back and left hip forward, so the hip bones are evenly facing the wall in front of you.
7. Take your tailbone in and the sitting bones down toward the backs of the knees.
8. Exhale; press the outer left foot firmly down.
9. Inhale; lift and broaden your chest.
10. Keeping the chest lifted, press the left outer heel firmly down and bend forward from the hips so your torso is as parallel to the floor as is possible, keeping space for your belly.

ENGAGING ACTIONS

1. Again, draw your right hip back and left hip forward.
2. Exhale; press the feet firmly down, especially the outer left foot.
3. Inhale; draw the sternum bone away from the navel; take the outer shoulders and elbows up toward the ceiling to lift and broaden the chest further.
4. Lift the kneecaps; firm your legs.
5. Soften your eyes, relax your face, and let the breath flow freely.

Stay for 5 breaths.

COMING OUT OF THE POSE

1. Press the feet firmly down and lead with the chest to come up.
2. Rotate the feet forward and release the arms to return to Utthita Hasta Padasana.

Repeat on the other side.

continued on next page

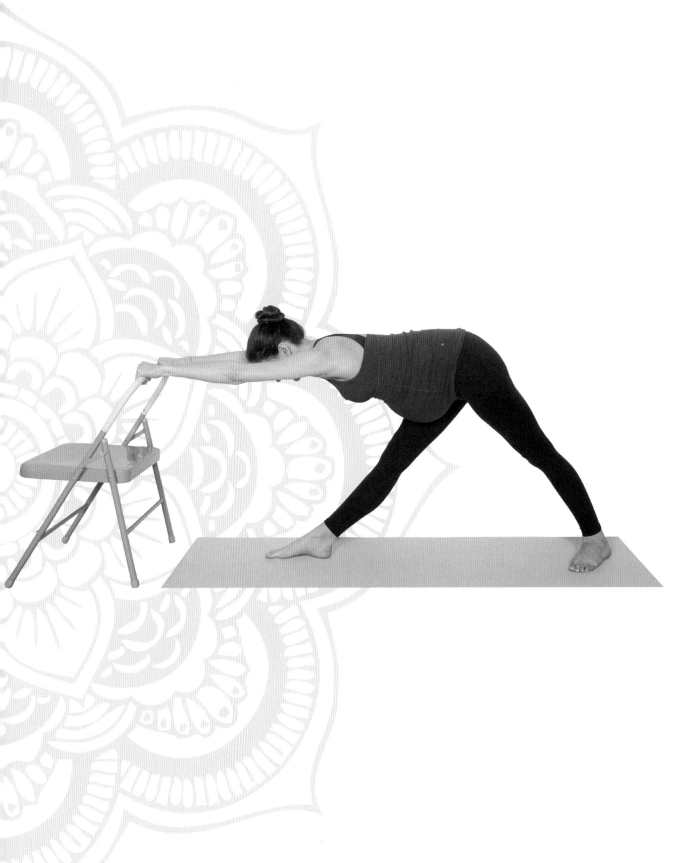

Variation: with chair

For more stability and elongation in the side body, you can practice with your hands on the backrest of a chair. It takes the balancing factor out of the pose.

1. Take a chair to the front of your sticky mat with the backrest facing toward you.
2. Stand in Tadasana facing the chair.
3. Step your left leg 3 to 3½ feet back and turn your left toes in to 80 degrees.
4. Place your hands on your hips.
5. Take the right hip back and the left hip forward, so the hip bones are evenly facing the wall in front of you.
6. Press the outer left foot firmly down.
7. Lift and broaden the chest.
8. Keeping the chest open; bend forward from your hips, and take your hands to the backrest of the chair.
9. Slide the chair away from you to elongate the sides of the body further.
10. Follow the same engaging actions as described above (except for taking the shoulders and elbows up toward the ceiling).

Coming out of the pose

1. Release your hands from the side rails of the chair and place your hands on your hips.
2. Press the feet firmly down and lead with the chest to come up.
3. Rotate the feet forward and release the arms to return to Utthita Hasta Padasana (p. 29).

Then repeat on the other side.

Prasarita Padottanasana: Concave

If you can't reach the
floor while keeping the
legs straight, try putting a
block under each hand.

Prasarita Padottanasana
Extended Intense Leg Stretch Pose

This pose soothes the nervous system, improves breathing, and rests the heart. It is helpful for improving digestion. It strengthens and stretches the legs, lengthens the spine, and opens the hips.

NOTE

In later stages of pregnancy if there is strain in the low back, back off or discontinue the pose altogether.

GETTING INTO THE POSE

1. Stand in Tadasana.
2. Step into Utthita Hasta Padasana (p. 29).
3. Be sure the outer feet are parallel to each other, toes turned in slightly.
4. Place the hands on the hips.
5. Spread your toes and balance evenly on your feet.
6. Exhale; from your outer hips, press your outer feet firmly down.
7. Inhale; lift and broaden the chest; lift the kneecaps up; straighten the legs fully.
8. Keeping the chest open, bend forward from your hips and place your hands on the floor or blocks; have your wrists directly under your shoulders and your hips in line with your ankles.

ENGAGING ACTIONS

1. Rotate the upper arms out; move the shoulders down away from the ears.
2. Exhale; from the outer hips press the outer feet firmly down.
3. Inhale; draw the sternum bone away from the navel and lift the kneecaps up; from the inner ankles lift the inner groins up.
4. Soften your face, relax your tongue, and let the breath flow freely.

DETAILS TO BE MINDFUL OF

To keep from overarching the back, draw the belly toward the spine.

Stay for 5–10 breaths.

continued on next page

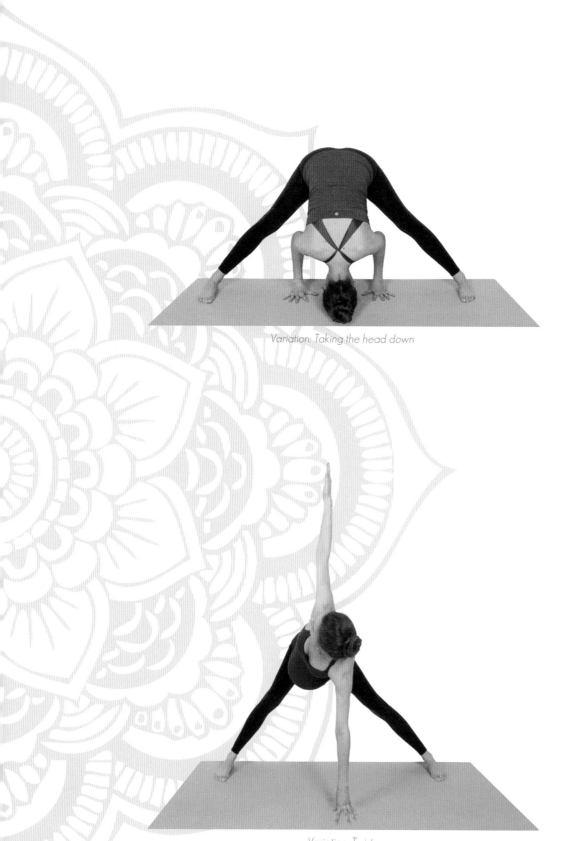

Variation: Taking the head down

Variation: Twist

Variation: Taking the head down

This variation should only be practiced in the earlier stages of pregnancy, to avoid compressing the belly.

1. From the concave version of the pose (p. 47), walk the hands between the legs as far as you can.
2. Bring the top of the head toward the floor.
3. Exhale; press the outer edges of the feet firmly into the floor; press the head down to the floor if it touches.
4. Inhale; lift the shoulders up, away from the ears, and lift the kneecaps up; lift the inner ankles up.
5. Soften your eyes, relax your face, and let the breath flow freely.

Stay for 5–10 breaths.

To come out of the pose

Walk your hands back out to the concave version of the pose so the wrists are directly under your shoulders, then press the feet firmly down and lead with the chest to come up.

Variation: Twist

This variation lengthens and strengthens the spine, bringing openness to the upper and mid back.

1. From the concave version of the pose (p. 47), take the left hand to the floor in front of you, centered between the feet.
2. Reach the right fingertips up toward the ceiling.
3. Keep taking the right shoulder back and the left chest forward to revolve the belly and chest.
4. Look up to the ceiling if it feels good.

Stay for 3–4 breaths.

Coming out of the pose

1. Bring the right hand back to the floor and repeat on the other side.
2. To come out of the pose, return to the concave version of the pose so the wrists are directly under your shoulders, then press the feet firmly down and lead with the chest to come up.

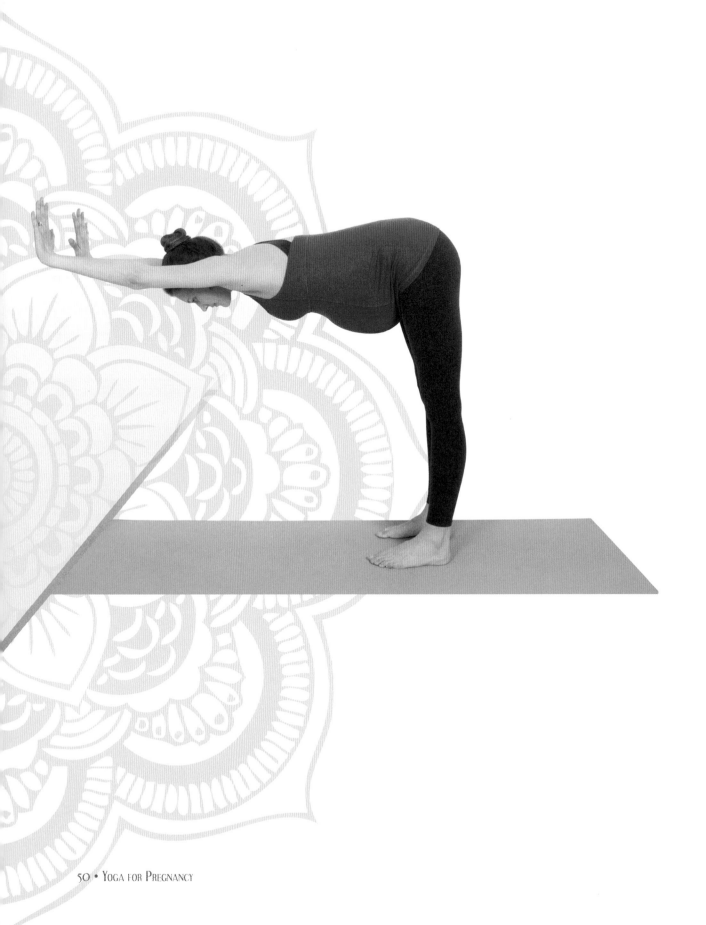

Ardha Uttanasana
Half Intense Stretch Pose

Practicing this pose brings length to your side ribs, providing added space for your baby to grow and for your breath. It also opens the chest, lengthens the hamstrings, and strengthens the legs. This is a variation of Uttanasana (next page) that can be practiced at all stages of pregnancy.

GETTING INTO THE POSE

1. Stand in Tadasana facing the wall.
2. Place your hands on the wall in line with your lower ribs and walk back so that your hips are in line with your shoulders and also in line with your ankles.
3. Have the ears in line with the arms.

ENGAGING ACTIONS

1. Straighten the arms and legs fully.
2. Rotate the upper arms out and the shoulders away from the ears.
3. Exhale; press the feet firmly down and press the hands into the wall.
4. Inhale; move the sternum bone toward the wall to lengthen the front of the body; lift the kneecaps up to firm your legs fully and extend the sitting bones toward the center of the room.
5. Soften your eyes, relax your face, and let the breath flow freely.

Stay for 5–10 breaths.

DETAILS TO BE MINDFUL OF

To prevent overarching the low back, draw your belly toward the spine.

COMING OUT OF THE POSE

1. Walk the feet toward the wall.
2. Press the feet firmly down and lead with the chest to come up.
3. Step the feet together to return to Tadasana.

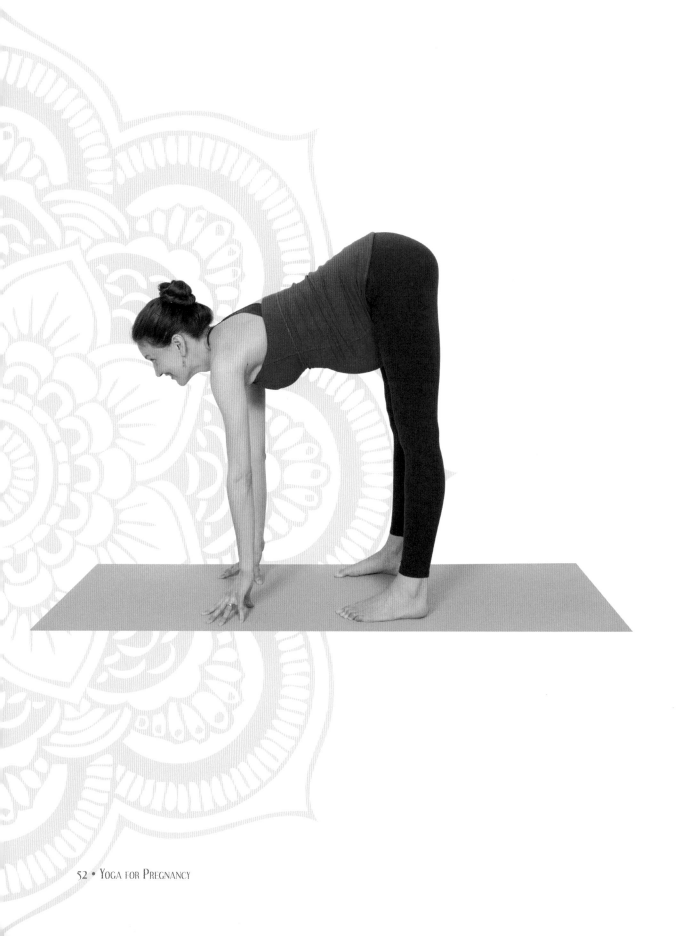

Uttanasana
Intense Stretch Pose

This pose provides an excellent way to open the hamstrings, strengthen the legs, and release the spine.

NOTE

The concave version of uttanasana as instructed here allows the belly to have space; folding forward as in the classic version of the pose is not recommended during pregnancy. Once the belly presses the thighs, practice Ardha Uttanasana (previous page) instead.

GETTING INTO THE POSE

1. Place two blocks on the tall height at the edge of your sticky mat, shoulder width apart.
2. Stand in Tadasana, half a foot back from the blocks.
3. Take your hands to your hips, spread your toes, and balance the weight evenly throughout your feet.
4. Exhale; press your feet into the floor.
5. Inhale; lift and broaden your chest.
6. Keep the sternum lifting away from your navel and bend forward from the hips to place your hands on the floor or the blocks. Take as much height as you need to keep your legs straight and your chest moving forward.
7. Move the blocks/hands so your wrists are directly under your shoulders.
8. Move the hips forward so they are in line with the ankles.

ENGAGING ACTIONS

1. Rotate the upper arms out, drawing the shoulders away from your ears.
2. Exhale; spread the weight throughout the feet.
3. Inhale; move the sternum forward, away from the belly.
4. Lift the kneecaps up and firm the legs fully.
5. Look forward and up.
6. Soften your eyes, relax your face, and let the breath flow freely.

DETAILS TO BE MINDFUL OF

- To keep from overarching your lower back, draw your belly toward the spine.
- It is important to keep the chest drawing forward and the shoulders back; it may be helpful to use blocks under your hands to support those actions.

Stay for 5–10 breaths.

COMING OUT OF THE POSE

Press the feet firmly down and lead with the chest to come up to Tadasana.

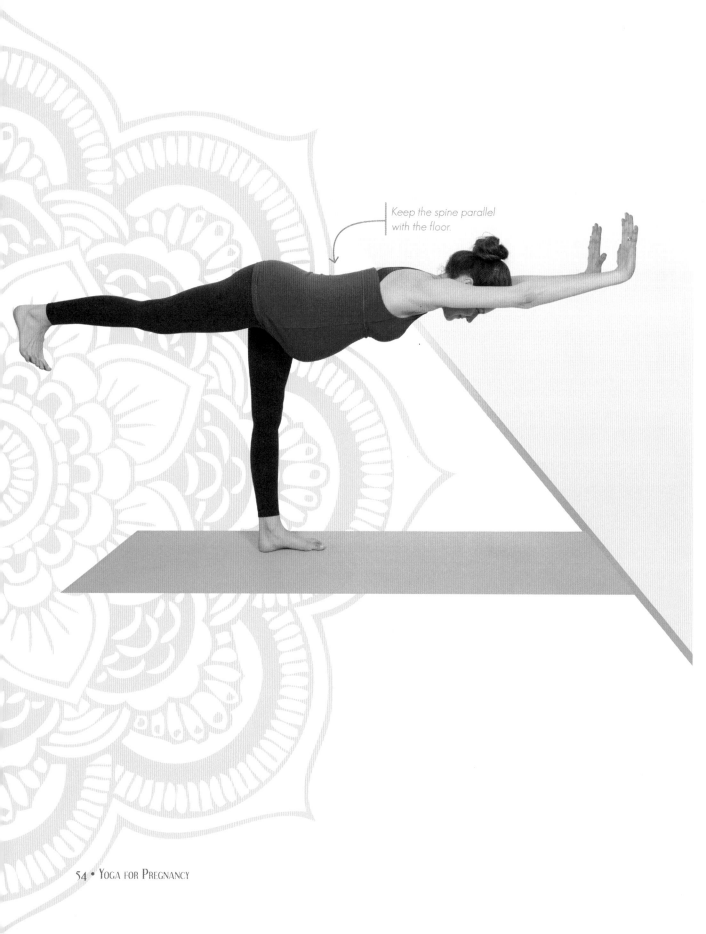

Keep the spine parallel with the floor.

Virabhadrasana III
Warrior III Pose

This modified version of Virabhadrasana III uses the wall for stability while still offering the same benefits as the classic pose. It activates circulation, generates heat, and instills inner and outer strength.

Getting into the pose

1. Stand in Tadasana facing the wall.
2. Place your hands on the wall in line with your lower ribs and walk back so that your hips are in line with your shoulders and also in line with your ankles.
3. Have the ears in line with your arms.
4. Straighten the arms and legs fully.
5. Draw the belly toward the spine.
6. Rotate the upper arms out and move the shoulders away from the ears.
7. Extend the sternum bone toward the wall to lengthen the whole front of your body; lift the kneecaps up.
8. Keeping all of these actions, lift the right leg up and back until it is parallel to the floor.

Engaging actions

1. Rotate the right hip down toward the floor so the buttock and hips are level.
2. Take the outer left hip back toward the center of the room.

3. Exhale; press the left foot firmly down and extend fully through the right inner heel and big toe mound; straighten the arms and legs fully.
4. Inhale; keep extending the sternum bone toward the wall.
5. Soften your eyes, relax your face, and let the breath flow freely.

Stay for 5 breaths.

Lower the right leg and repeat on the other side.

Coming out of the pose

1. Walk the feet toward the wall.
2. Press the feet firmly down and lead with the chest to come up to Tadasana.

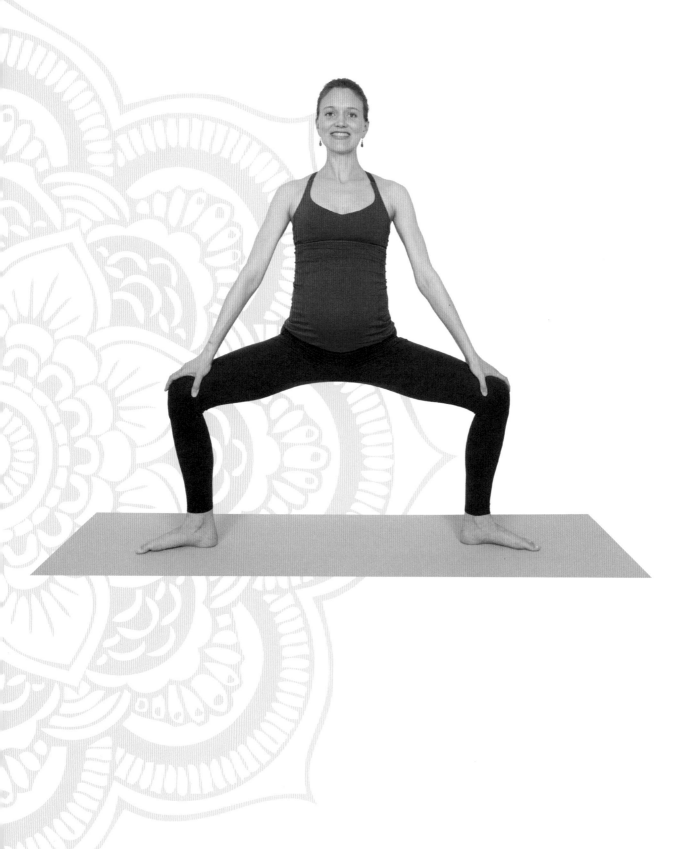

Half Squat

Practicing squatting is an amazingly beneficial preparation for labor. Squats open the hips, stretch the calves, and encourage baby to get into a good position for labor. Also, being able to squat during labor can be invaluable in helping labor progress.

NOTE

If baby is not head down at the end of pregnancy (after about 34 weeks), discontinue this pose.

This is a great pose to practice your Kegels (p. 161).

GETTING INTO THE POSE

1. Stand with your feet just wider than hip width apart and turn the toes out.
2. Bend your knees and place your hands on your thighs.

ENGAGING ACTIONS

1. Draw the tailbone in and the sitting bones down.
2. Draw the shoulders back and down.
3. Exhale; press the heels firmly down.
4. Lift the pubic bone toward the navel.
5. Inhale; lift and broaden the chest.
6. Soften your eyes, relax your face, and let the breath flow freely.

Stay here for 5–10 breaths.

COMING OUT OF THE POSE

Straighten the legs and rest a moment.

Repeat a few times.

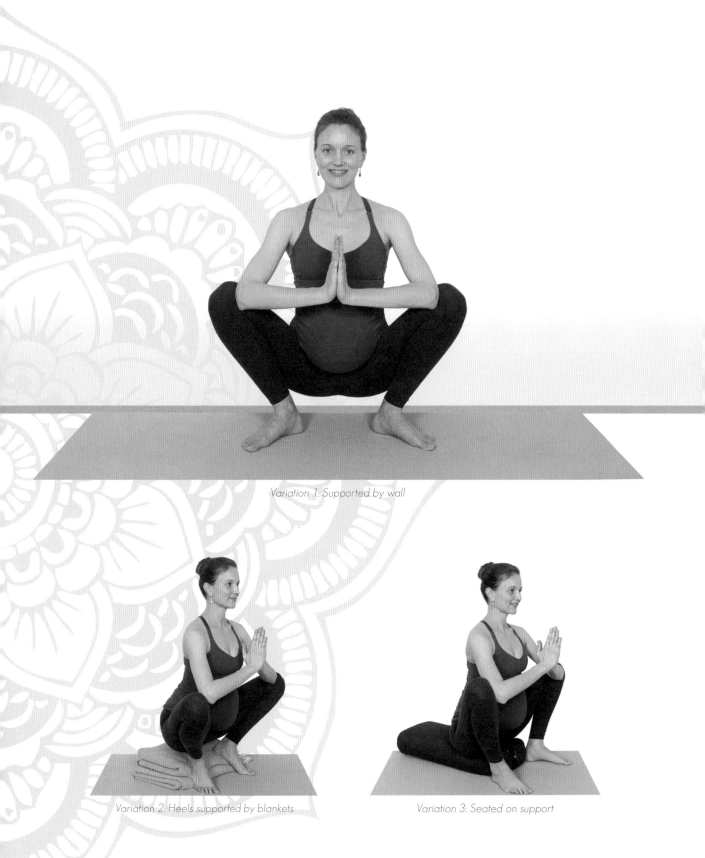

Variation 1: Supported by wall

Variation 2: Heels supported by blankets

Variation 3: Seated on support

Full Squat

Full Squats have even more of the important benefits of Half Squats (previous page). They are extremely valuable throughout pregnancy and also during labor.

NOTE

This is a great pose to practice your Kegels (p. 161).

VARIATION 1: SUPPORTED BY WALL

1. Stand with the heels a few inches away from the wall and the buttock lightly touching the wall; have the feet wider than hip width apart and the feet turned out slightly.
2. Bend the knees and come into a squat; adjust your feet if needed so you are supported by the wall.
3. Place your elbows to the inside of the thighs, press your hands together, and press the knees away to widen the thighs.
4. Draw the tailbone in.
5. Draw the shoulders back and down.
6. Exhale; press the heels firmly down, especially the inner heels.
7. Draw the pubic bone toward the navel.
8. Inhale, lift and broaden the chest.
9. Soften your eyes, relax your face, and let the breath flow freely.

Stay for 5–10 breaths.

COMING OUT OF THE POSE

To come out of the pose, take the hands to the floor, step the feet wide apart with outer edges of the feet parallel; press the feet firmly down and lead with the chest to come up.

VARIATION 2: HEELS SUPPORTED BY BLANKETS

1. Stand with your heels on two blankets in Basic Fold, feet wider than hip width apart and turned out slightly.
2. Bend your knees and come into a squat.
3. Follow instructions 3–9 from Variation 1.

Stay for 5–10 breaths.

COMING OUT OF THE POSE

To come out of the pose, take the hands to the floor, step the feet wide apart with outer edges of the feet parallel; press the feet firmly down and lead with the chest to come up.

VARIATION 3: SEATED ON SUPPORT

1. Sit on a bolster or blankets and follow instructions 3–9 from Variation 1.

Stay for 5–10 breaths.

COMING OUT OF THE POSE

Extend your legs straight out in Dandasana.

continued on next page

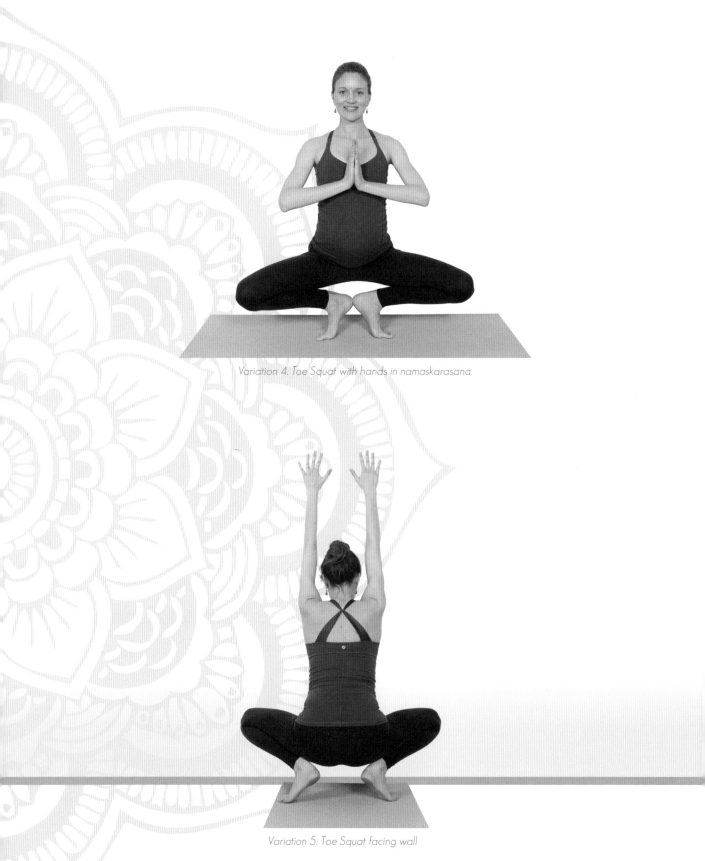

Variation 4: Toe Squat with hands in namaskarasana

Variation 5: Toe Squat facing wall

Variation 4: Toe Squat

1. Come into a squat position with your toe pads and toes on the floor and the heels together.
2. Place the hands onto a tall block, on the thighs, or in Namaskarasana (as shown).
3. Draw the shoulders back and down.
4. Draw the tailbone in.
5. Exhale; press the heels together and take the knees wide apart.
6. Inhale; lift and broaden the chest.
7. Soften your eyes, relax your face, and let the breath flow freely.

Stay for 5–10 breaths.

Coming out of the Pose

To come out of the pose, take the hands to the floor and step the feet wide apart with outer edges of the feet parallel; press the feet firmly down and lead with the chest to come up.

Variation 5: Toe Squat facing wall

This variation is more restful and also helps open the shoulders.

1. Come into Toe Squat with your feet a few inches away from the wall.
2. Walk the hands up the wall; rest your forehead and knees against the wall for support.
3. Follow instructions 3–7 from Variation 4.

Stay for 5–10 breaths.

Coming out of the Pose

To come out of the pose, take the hands to the floor and step the feet wide apart with outer edges of the feet parallel; press the feet firmly down and lead with the chest to come up.

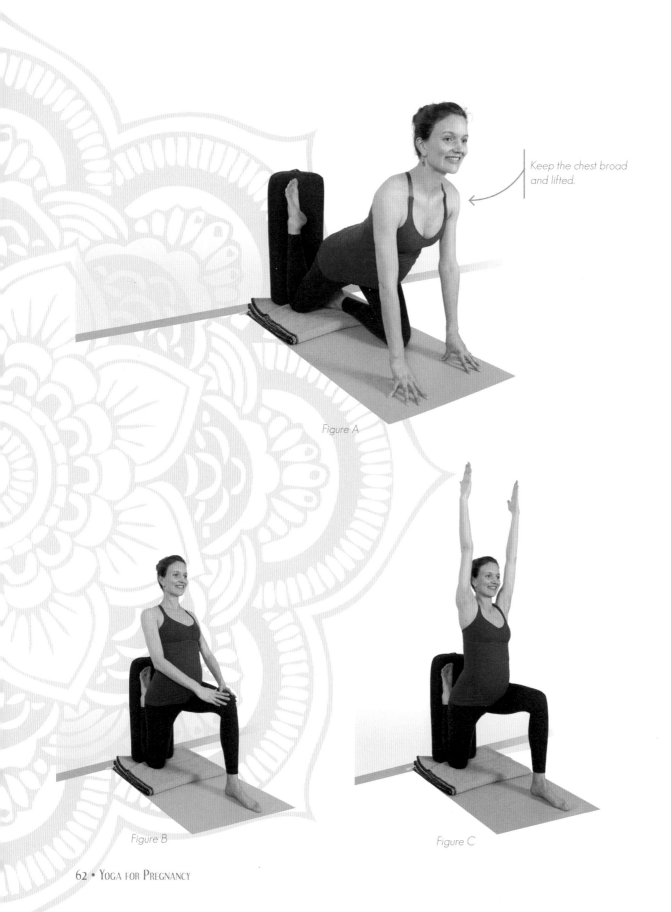

Keep the chest broad
and lifted.

Figure A

Figure B

Figure C

Half Lunge at Wall

This pose opens the hip flexors and stretches the quadriceps muscles; this in turn can alleviate low back pain, which often stems from these areas being tight.

NOTE

The intensity of this pose offers a good opportunity to prepare for labor; see if you can use the breath to quiet the mind and become fully present with the powerful, opening physical sensations.

If you experience any knee strain in this pose, try adjusting where the knee is pressing into the floor by shifting it slightly forward or back (micro movements). Also try pressing the little toes into the bolster. If that doesn't resolve it, back off or discontinue the pose altogether.

GETTING INTO THE POSE

1. Place a blanket by a wall and place a bolster on top of it (this can be done without a bolster if you don't have one).
2. Kneel on the blanket and have the outer right thigh against the bolster; rotate toward the center of the room and take the right shin up the bolster so the right big toe points straight up to the ceiling.
3. Place the hands on the floor; the left shin is on the floor and the left knee points away from your midline to accommodate space for your belly.
4. Draw the tailbone in; draw the shoulders back and down.
5. Draw the pubic bone toward the navel; lift and broaden the chest.
6. Stay here in this variation if you feel a good stretch *(Figure A)*.
7. If you'd like more stretch, place the left foot on the floor, taking the leg out to the side as needed to maintain space for your belly.
8. Line up the center of the knee with the center of the foot, keeping the knee in line with the ankle. Place your hands on your thigh *(Figure B)*.
9. Repeat actions #4 and #5.
10. Stay here in this variation if you feel a good stretch.
11. If you'd like more stretch, take your back closer to the wall and extend the arms up.
12. Draw the tailbone in.
13. Roll the upper arms in and keep extending the chest away from the navel *(Figure C)*.

DETAILS TO BE MINDFUL OF

- To keep from overarching the back, draw the front ribs into the back body and the tailbone in; lift the pubic bone and the lower belly up.
- Keep the head in line with the spine.

Stay for 5–10 breaths.

COMING OUT OF THE POSE

1. If the hands are up, take them back to the floor.
2. Take the left shin back to the floor. Take the right shin away from the wall.

Repeat on the other side.

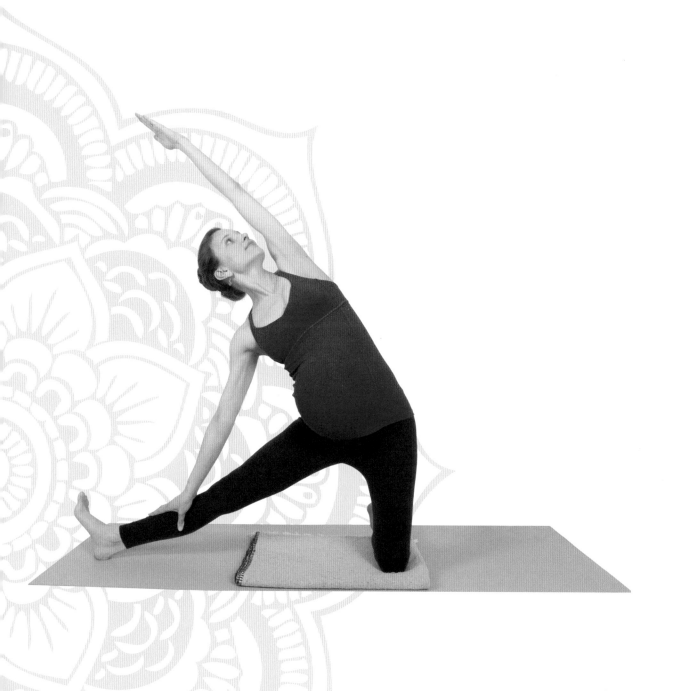

Parighasana
Gate Latch Pose

This pose opens the sides of the body, making more space for baby to grow and for your breath.

Getting into the Pose

1. Spread a blanket on your mat in Open Fold (p. 6).
2. Come to kneeling and take the hands to the hips.
3. Take the right foot out to the right side and an inch or two back from in line with the knee.
4. Straighten the right leg and flex the right foot, pressing out firmly through the inner heel and big toe mound.
5. Rotate the right thigh from inner to outer; your right knee and toes should be pointing straight up toward the ceiling.
6. Keeping the chest facing forward, press the left shin and the top of the left foot down.
7. Bend at the right hip crease and bring the right hand to the right shin.
8. Take your left hand to your left hip.
9. Take your left elbow and shoulder back and your right chest and right buttock forward.
10. Keeping that rotation, extend your left arm to the left and reach through your fingertips, keeping the wrist in line with the shoulder.
11. Again, press the left shin and the top of the left foot down.
12. Turn the left palm up and reach the arm over the head like in Parsvakonasana (p. 37); rotate the upper arm in and reach actively through the fingertips.

Engaging Actions

1. Draw the tailbone in.
2. Draw the shoulders away from the ears.
3. Exhale; press down into the left shin and the top of the left foot.
4. Inhale; take your chest away from your navel and extend strongly through your left fingertips.
5. Rotate your belly and chest up to the ceiling and look up to the inside of the arm if that feels good, or you can keep your gaze focused straight ahead.
6. Soften your eyes, relax your face, and let the breath flow freely.

Stay for 5–10 breaths.

Coming out of the Pose

1. Rotate your gaze back to center.
2. Lower your left arm to shoulder height.
3. Press down into the left shin and reach through the left fingertips to come up.

Repeat on the other side.

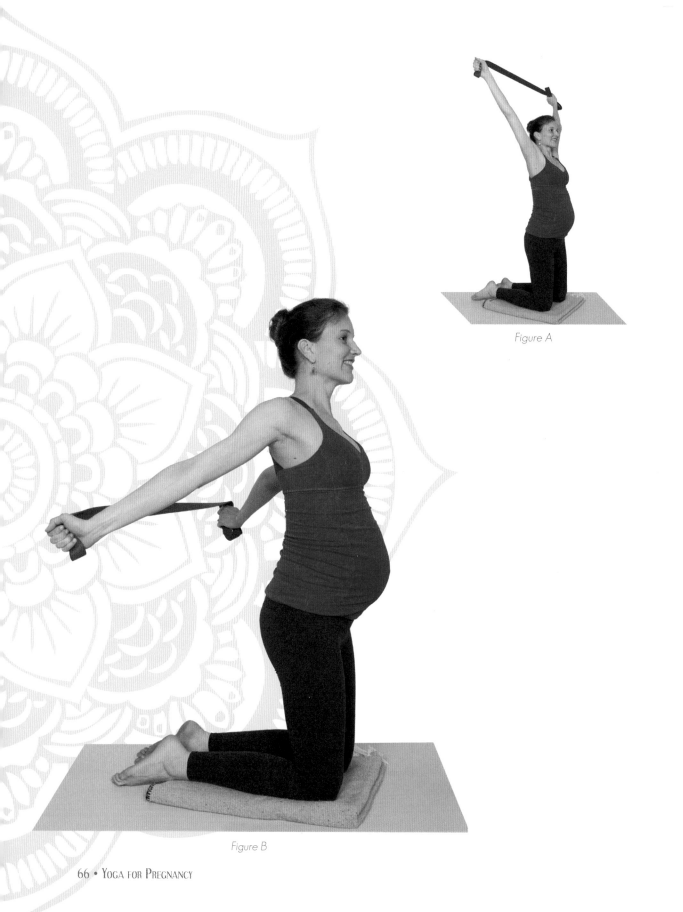

Figure A

Figure B

Kneeling Chest Opener

This is a great pose to open the chest and release tension in the neck and shoulders. It is also a wonderful postpartum pose to counteract back tension from constantly rounding forward while holding baby (especially if you are breastfeeding).

Getting into the pose

1. Place a blanket on your sticky mat in Open Fold (p. 6).
2. Kneel on the blanket and take hold of a belt with your hands a foot or so wider than shoulder width.

Engaging actions

1. Draw the tailbone in and the sitting bones down.
2. Exhale; press the shins down.
3. Inhale; lift and broaden the chest; extend the arms over head (*Figure A*).
4. Pull the hands away from one another.
5. With your next exhalation, take the arms behind you and down toward the floor (*Figure B*). Keep pulling the hands away from one another.
6. With your next inhalation extend the arms up overhead again.
7. Continue steps #5 and #6 for 10–15 breaths, coordinating the inhales and exhales with your movements.
8. If you feel areas that are particularly tight, pause there and take a few breaths.
9. Soften your eyes, relax your face, and let the breath flow freely.

Repeat for 10–15 breaths.

Coming out of the pose

Release the belt and sit for a moment, enjoying the new spaciousness in your upper back, shoulders, and neck.

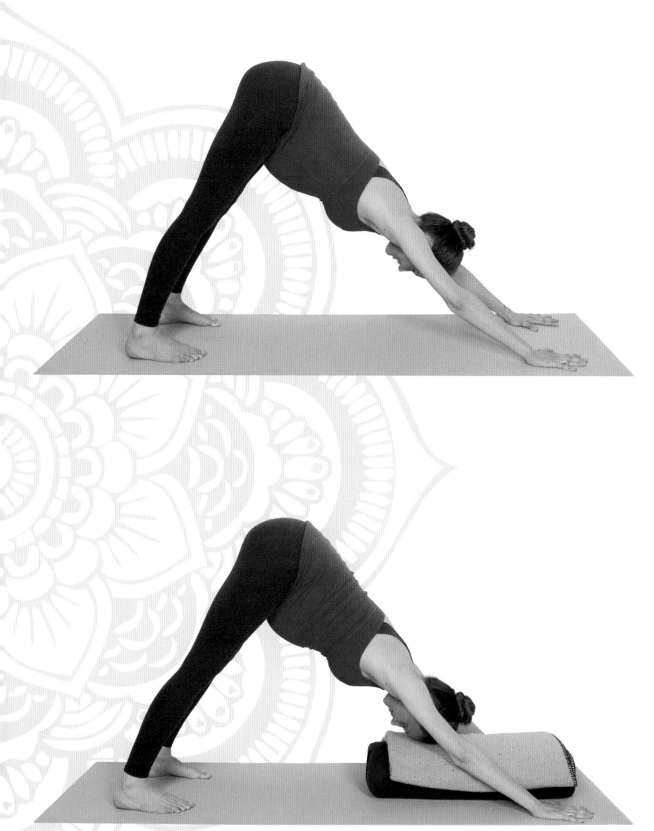

Variation: Head supported

Adho Mukha Svanasana

Downward Facing Dog Pose

This foundational pose has numerous benefits. It brings length and strength to the spine, eases back pain, and also firms the arms and legs. Adho Mukha Svanasana is an energizing and relaxing pose that helps relieve stress and mild depression. It can also help lower blood pressure, especially when done with the head supported.

Note

In later stages of pregnancy, take your feet wider apart to accommodate your belly.

Coming into the pose

1. Start on your hands and knees.
2. Slide the knees two inches back from the hips.
3. Spread the fingers wide and press the mounds of the pointer fingers firmly down.
4. Rotate the upper arms out and take the shoulders away from the ears.
5. Draw the sternum bone forward.
6. Look forward.
7. Keeping the chest and head forward, turn the toes under.
8. Take a deep inhalation and exhale to lift the hips up.
9. Release your head and neck.

Engaging actions

1. Rotate the upper arms out and press into the mounds of the fingers.
2. Inhale; lift the sitting bones and the outer hips higher.
3. Lift up and out of the shoulders.
4. Exhale; keep the hips lifted; press the front of the thighs back toward the back of the thighs; press the inner thighs back so the legs are super firm.
5. If you can keep your hips fully lifted, press the heels toward the floor.

6. Soften your eyes, relax your face, and let the breath flow freely.

Stay for 5–10 breaths.

Coming out of the pose

1. Come back to hands and knees.
2. Lower into Adho Mukha Virasana (p. 107) and rest for a few breaths.

There are several variations of this pose that are nice for later stages of pregnancy and when tired:

Variation: Head supported

Support the head with a bolster. Make sure to keep lifting the shoulders away from the bolster and keep the neck long. Keep the arms straight. If you need more height, add a blanket or two on top of the bolster. Conversely, you can take height away if the neck is feeling compressed in any way.

continued on next page

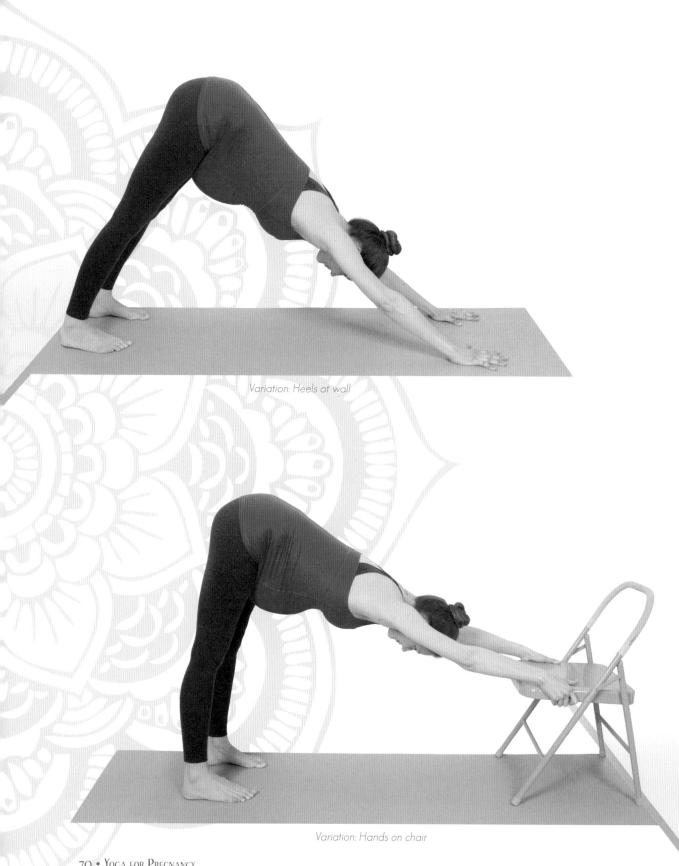

Variation: Heels at wall

Variation: Hands on chair

VARIATION: HEELS AT WALL

On your hands and knees, align yourself so that the tips of your toes are just touching the wall, ankles in line with your knees. Proceed into the classic pose; when you lift your hips your heels will be pressing into the wall, and the pads of the toes will be on the floor. Take your heels down to the floor, as long as you can keep your hips lifted.

VARIATION: HANDS ON CHAIR

Place a chair at the wall on your sticky mat with the seat facing the middle of the room and the back legs of the chair against the wall. Hold on to the outer edges of the seat and proceed as with the classic pose.

VARIATION: HANDS AT WALL

(not shown)

On your hands and knees, align yourself so that your hands are right up against the wall. The thumbs and tips of the pointer fingers are touching the wall. Proceed into the classic pose, pressing into the wall for extra stability and length in the arms.

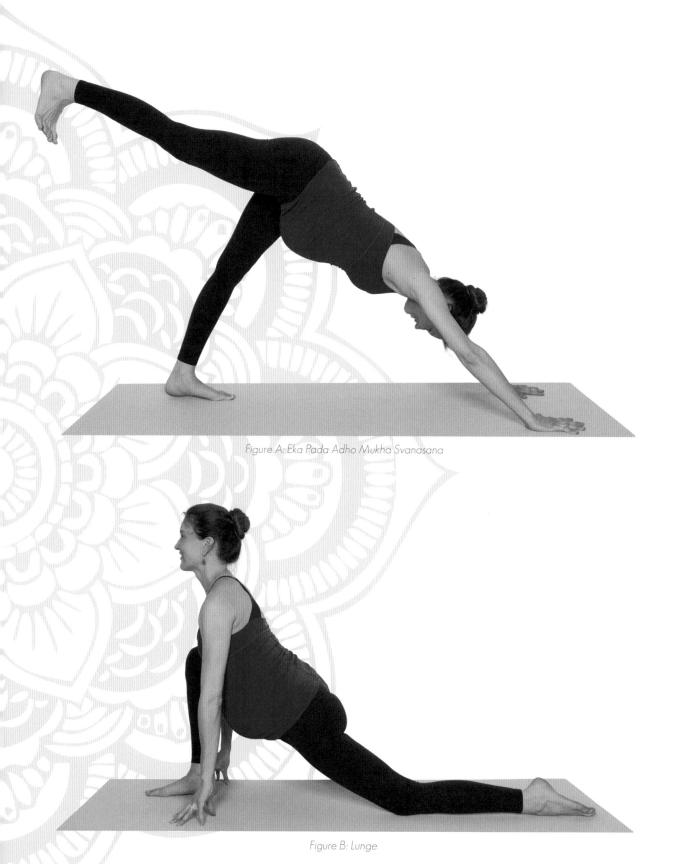

Figure A: Eka Pada Adho Mukha Svanasana

Figure B: Lunge

Eka Pada Adho Mukha Svanasana & Lunge

One Foot Downward Facing Dog Pose • Lunge

Lunges strengthen the legs and open the hip flexors. They are extremely helpful both for people who are very active and athletic and for those who do a lot of sitting.

Note

Late in pregnancy, coming into a lunge from Eka Pada Adho Mukha Svanasana will not be possible; instead, start on your hands and knees, then step the right foot forward.

Getting into the Pose

1. Start in Adho Mukha Svanasana (previous page).
2. Extend the right leg up and back.
3. Rotate the right hip down toward the floor and the left hip back toward the wall to keep the low back stable; pause here in Eka Pada Adho Mukha Svanasana for a few breaths *(Figure A)*.
4. Bend the right knee and take the right heel to the buttock.
5. Swing your right foot forward and place your foot on the floor as far away from the midline as you need to accommodate your belly; check to make sure that your right knee is in line with the center of the foot and ankle.
6. Lower your left knee to the ground *(Figure B)*.

Engaging Actions

1. Draw your tailbone in.
2. Take the outer right hip back toward the wall behind you.
3. Rotate the upper arms out and draw the shoulders away from the ears.
4. Exhale; move forward and deepen the stretch in your hip flexor.
5. Inhale; lift the pubic bone toward the navel; draw the sternum bone away from the navel.
6. Soften your eyes, relax your face, and let the breath flow freely.

Details to be Mindful of

- It is important to keep the chest open and the shoulders back; it may be helpful to use blocks under your hands to support these actions.
- Keep the knee in line with the center of the foot and directly above the ankle; the knee should be bent at a 90-degree angle.

Stay for 5 breaths.

Coming out of the Pose

Place the hands flat on the ground and step your left foot back into Adho Mukha Svanasana.

Repeat on the other side.

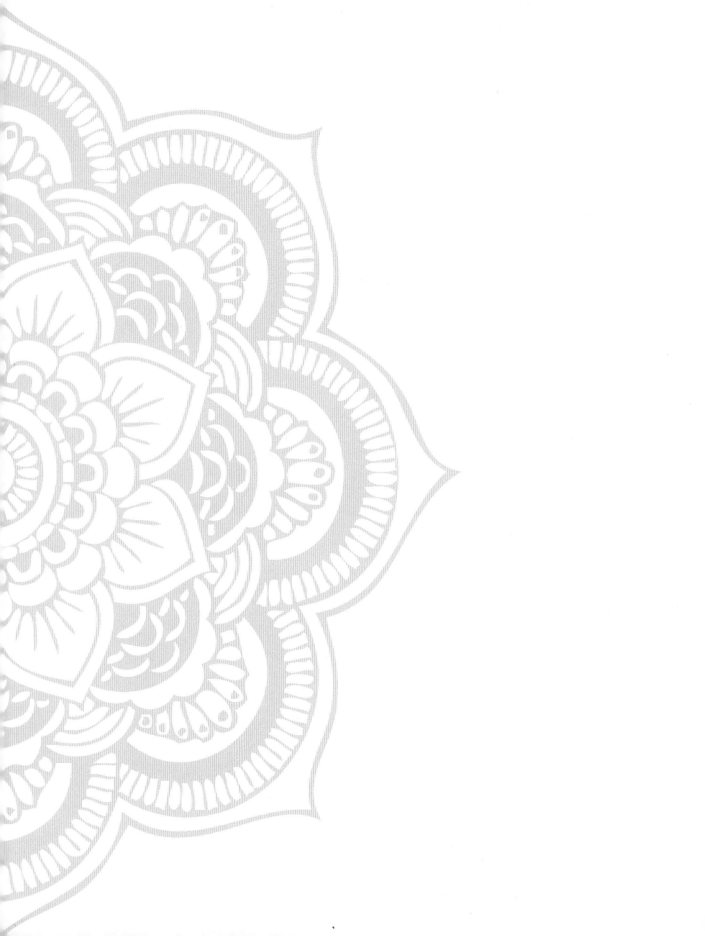

SEATED POSES

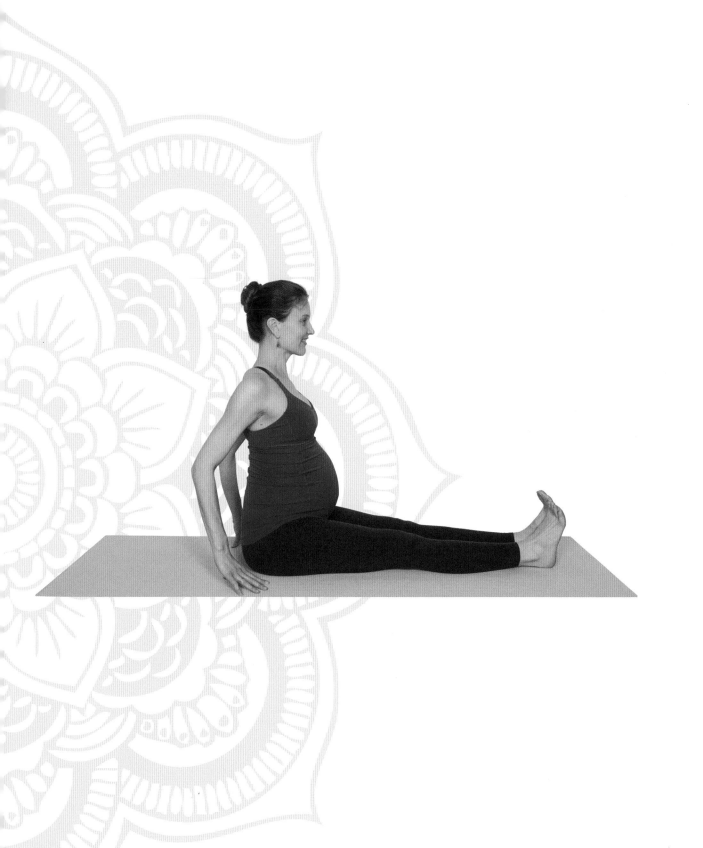

Dandasana
Staff Pose

Dandasana is like the Tadasana of the seated poses. It is a stabilizing pose; after each seated posture it is helpful to come to Dandasana before moving to the next pose in order to open the backs of the knees and regain balance.

Getting into the pose

1. Sit on the floor with your legs straight forward, big toes pointing straight up; the legs are as close together as you can have them while accommodating your belly.
2. Place your fingertips or palms on the floor by your sides and a little behind your shoulders.

Engaging actions

1. Rotate the upper arms out; draw the shoulders away from your ears.
2. From the back of the knees, press firmly out through your heels and extend through the big toe mounds.
3. Exhale; press the hands down and press the head of the thigh bones down; firm the legs completely.
4. Inhale; lift and broaden the chest; lift even the tips of the ears up.
5. Soften your eyes, relax your face, and let the breath flow freely.

Details to be mindful of

Your torso should be perpendicular to the floor; if necessary, sit up on a blanket or two to achieve this.

Stay for 5–10 breaths.

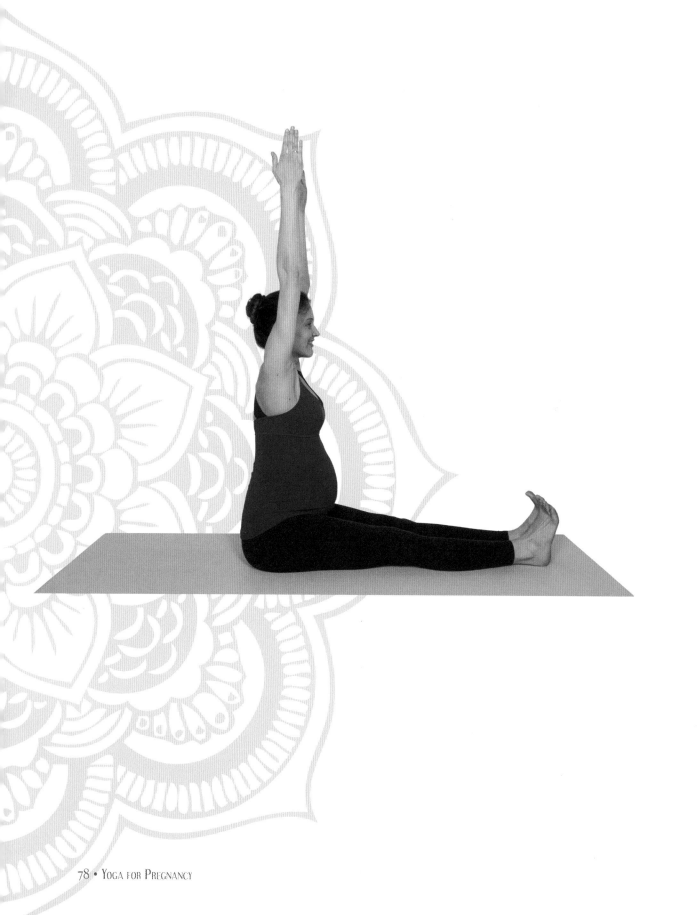

Urdhva Hasta Dandasana
Upward Hand Staff Pose

This is a variation of Dandasana. In this version of the pose the sides of the body and spine are opened and the arms are strengthened.

GETTING INTO THE POSE

From Dandasana, extend your arms up over the head with the wrists shoulder width apart and palms facing each other.

ENGAGING ACTIONS

1. Keeping the arms parallel to each other, rotate the upper arms in toward your midline.
2. Draw the inner shoulder blades down.
3. Exhale; press the head of the thigh bones down.
4. Inhale; lift and broaden the chest; extend fully through the fingertips.
5. Soften your eyes, relax your face, and let the breath flow freely.

Stay for 5–10 breaths.

COMING OUT OF THE POSE

Release the arms and return to Dandasana.

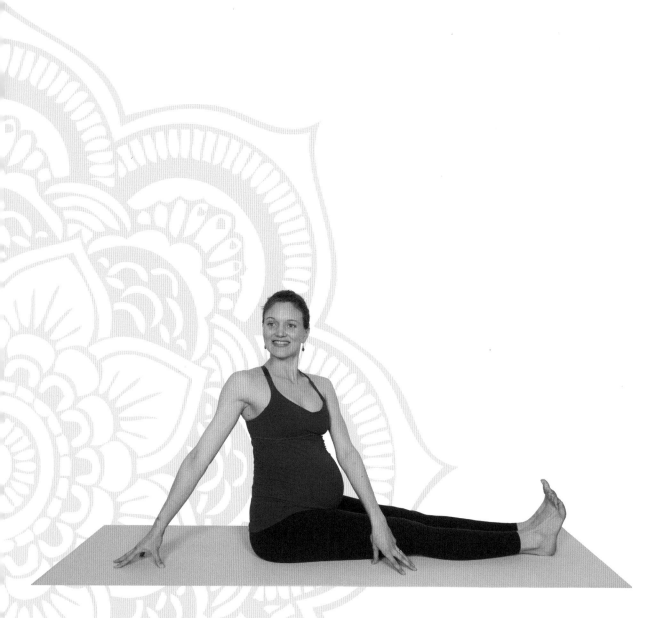

Parivrtta Dandasana
Revolved Staff Pose

This variation of Dandasana provides a twisting action for the spine. The belly remains open, making it a suitable twist during pregnancy.

Getting into the pose

1. Sit in Dandasana, then extend your arms into Urdhva Hasta Dandasana.
2. Bring your right fingertips to the floor behind you.
3. Take your left hand to the outside of your right thigh.

Engaging actions

1. Rotate the upper arms out, drawing the shoulders away from your ears.
2. Exhale; press the hands down and press the head of the thigh bones down.
3. Inhale; lift and broaden the chest.
4. Keeping the chest lifted, exhale and revolve the belly and chest to the right, letting your head follow.
5. With each inhalation lift the chest more to lengthen the spine upward; with each exhalation see if you can rotate more into the twist.
6. Soften your eyes, relax your face, and let the breath flow freely.

Stay for 5–10 breaths.

Coming out of the pose

1. Extend the arms overhead into Urdhva Hasta Dandasana.
2. Release the arms and return to Dandasana.

Repeat on the other side.

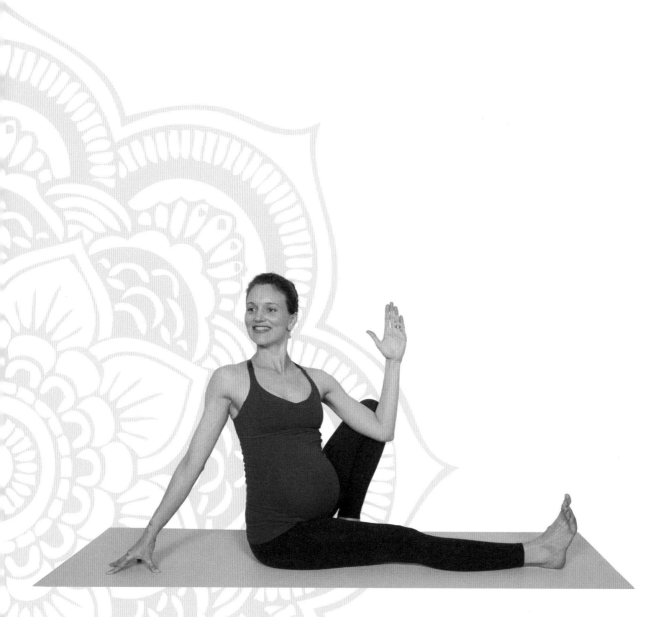

Marichyasana I
Marichi's Pose

Marichyasana I strengthens and stretches the spine. It also opens the shoulders and relieves back discomfort.

NOTE

Like Bharadvajasana (p. 91), this is a twist where the belly is not compressed and is therefore fine during pregnancy.

If you are able to sit on the floor with the spine fully lifted and perpendicular to the floor, then you can do this pose without a blanket. If it is hard to keep the chest lifted, sit on two blankets.

GETTING INTO THE POSE

1. Start in Dandasana, sitting on one blanket in Basic Fold.
2. Bend the left knee and take the heel in line with the sitting bone (or as far out away from the midline as necessary to make space for your belly); see that the knee and ankle are in line with one another.
3. Extend firmly out through the right inner heel and big toe mound.
4. Extend your arms straight up like in Urdhva Hasta Dandasana (p. 79).
5. Bring your right fingertips to the floor or blankets behind you.
6. Lift and broaden the chest and reach through your left fingertips.
7. Keeping the chest lifted, take your left elbow to the inner left thigh.

ENGAGING ACTIONS

1. Rotate the upper arms out, draw the shoulders down.
2. Exhale; press the head of the right thigh bone down; press the left foot down; press the right hand down.
3. Inhale; lift and broaden the chest.
4. Exhale; keeping the chest lifted, press the left elbow and inner thigh together and revolve the belly and chest to the right, letting your head follow.
5. With each inhalation keep lifting the chest; with each exhalation revolve further to the right.
6. Soften your eyes, relax your face, and let the breath flow freely.

Stay for 5–10 breaths.

COMING OUT OF THE POSE

Release the arms and leg to return to Dandasana.

Repeat on the other side.

Pull back on the belt; draw the shoulders down; lift and broaden the chest.

Janu Sirsasana
Head to Knee Pose

This pose opens the hips, chest, and hamstrings. It also creates strength in the upper back.

NOTE

While pregnant, only do the concave version of this pose as described below. The classic version of the pose compresses the belly, which is contraindicated during pregnancy.

GETTING INTO THE POSE

1. Start in Dandasana, sitting on one blanket in Basic Fold.
2. Place a belt beyond your feet, with the ends of the belt toward you.
3. Take your right hand to your inner right knee; use your hand to bend and slide your knee out to the right side.
4. With your right hand, grip under your right ankle and take your right foot to the inner left thigh with the heel as close in toward the perineum as possible.
5. Flex both the feet, pressing through the inner heels and big toe mounds.
6. Be sure that the left foot and center of the left knee are pointing straight up to the ceiling.
7. Rotate the left hip back and the right hip forward so that the hips are even.
8. Take hold of the belt with each hand; walk your hands down the belt as far as you can while keeping your arms and legs straight and maintaining enough room for baby.

ENGAGING ACTIONS

1. Rotate the upper arms out; draw the shoulders down away from your ears.
2. Exhale; press the outer right knee and the inner left thigh down.
3. Inhale; lift and broaden the chest; pull back on the belt to lift the side chest up.
4. Soften your eyes, relax your face, and let the breath flow freely.

Stay for 5–10 breaths.

COMING OUT OF THE POSE

Release the belt and return to Dandasana.

Repeat on the other side.

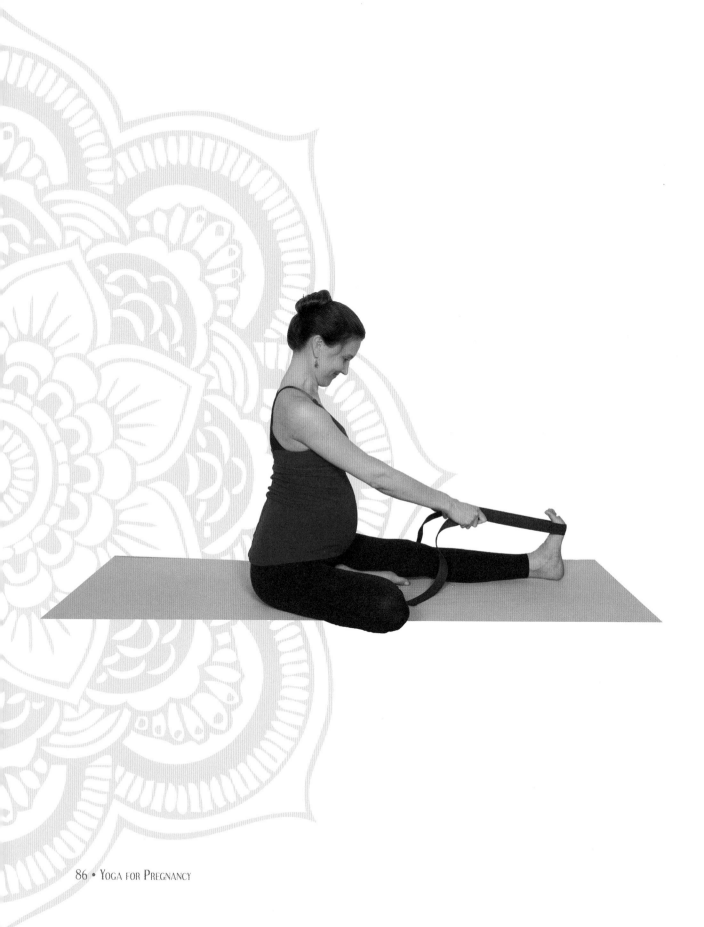

Maha Mudra
The Great Seal Pose

This is a great pose for expanding the ribs, which gives more room for baby to grow as well as more room for your breath. It is also a helpful aid for nausea and digestion. The practice of bowing the head down to the heart, as done in this pose, is quieting to the mind.

NOTE

In the classic version of this pose there are three bandhas ("bandha" can be translated as a hold, block, or seal). Only two of these should be performed during pregnancy: Mula Bandha (lifting of the pelvic floor), and Jalandhara Bandha (chin lock or seal, with the head drawn down). The third bandha, Uddiyana Bandha (drawing in and up of the abdomen), is not to be performed during pregnancy.

GETTING INTO THE POSE

1. Start in Dandasana, sitting on one blanket in Basic Fold.
2. Place a belt beyond your feet, with the ends of the belt toward you.
3. Move your right leg and arms into the same position as Janu Sirsasana (previous page, steps 3 and 4 in "Getting into the pose").
4. Flex both the feet, pressing through the inner heels and big toe mounds.
5. Be sure that the left foot and center of the knee are pointing straight up to the ceiling.
6. Rotate the right hip forward and left hip back so that the front of the hips are even.
7. Take hold of the belt with each hand; walk your hands down the belt as much as you can while keeping your arms and legs straight and having enough room for baby.

ENGAGING ACTIONS

1. Rotate the upper arms out, draw the shoulders away from your ears.
2. Exhale; press the outer right knee and the root of the left thigh down.

3. Inhale; lift and broaden the chest; pull back on the belt to lift the side chest up. Lift your forearms up to the ceiling.
4. Keeping your chest broad and lifted, lower the chin down until the chin meets your chest, and rest your chin in the notch between the collarbones. This is Jalandhara Bandha.
5. Fully relax your head, forehead, tongue, and especially your throat.
6. Exhale all the air out of your lungs and take a deep full breath in.
7. As you breathe in, lift the pelvic floor up in a Kegel-like action, and hold it for your entire inhalation; this is Mula Bandha.
8. When you are ready to exhale, release Mula Bandha.

Continue with your breath and Mula Bandha on the inhalations in this pose for a few more breaths, ending with an exhalation.

NOTE

If you are not able to take your head to your chest and keep your chest and spine lifted, then practice this pose instead with your head looking up toward the ceiling. This encourages your chest to remain lifted. Look upward for each inhalation and look straight forward as you exhale, repeating with your breath.

COMING OUT OF THE POSE

Lift your head, release the grip of the belt, and return to Dandasana.

Repeat on the other side.

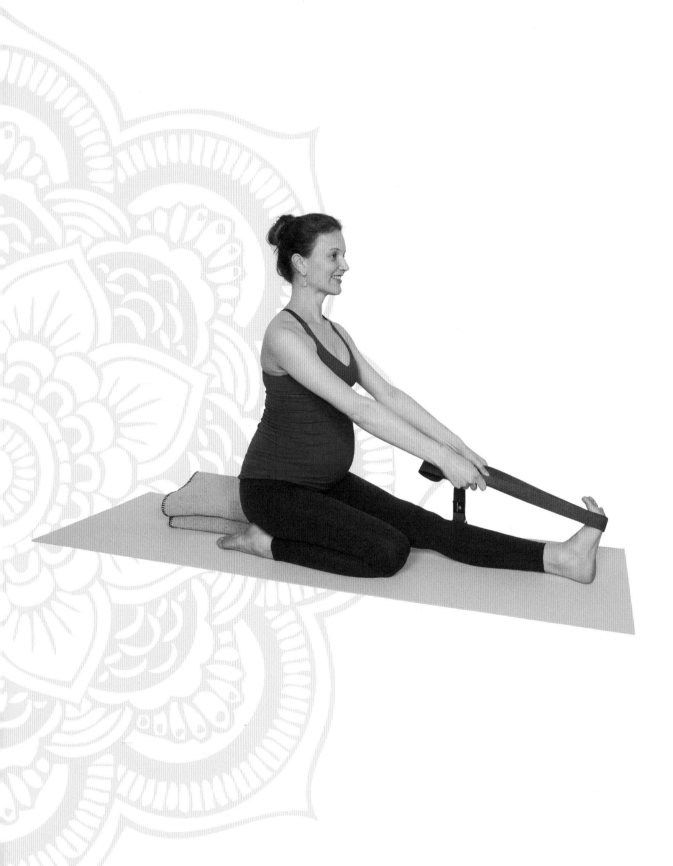

Triang Mukhaipada Paschimottanasana
Three Limbed One Foot Intense Stretch of the West Pose

This pose stretches the legs and ankles and opens the chest. It is strengthening to the upper back and arms.

NOTE

While pregnant, only do the concave version of this pose as described below. The classic version of the pose compresses the belly, which is contraindicated during pregnancy.

GETTING INTO THE POSE

1. Start in Dandasana, sitting on two blankets in Narrow Fold (p. 6).
2. Place a belt beyond your feet, with the ends of the belt toward you.
3. Sit on the left edge of the blanket and fold your right leg back as in Virasana (p. 105); point your big toe straight back and roll the calf out away from the midline; spread and press the toes down; especially press the little toe down.
4. Place the belt around the ball of the left foot and flex the foot, pressing through the inner heel and big toe mound.
5. Be sure that the left foot and center of the knee are pointing straight up to the ceiling.
6. Walk your hands down the belt as much as you can while keeping your arms and legs straight and having enough room for baby.

ENGAGING ACTIONS

1. Rotate the upper arms out, drawing the shoulders away from your ears.
2. Exhale; press the right toes down and press the head of the left thigh bone down.
3. Inhale; lift and broaden the chest; lift even the tips of the ears up. Pull back on the belt to lift and open the chest further.
4. Soften your eyes, relax your face, and let the breath flow freely.

Stay for 5–10 breaths.

COMING OUT OF THE POSE

Release the belt and return to Dandasana.

Repeat on the other side.

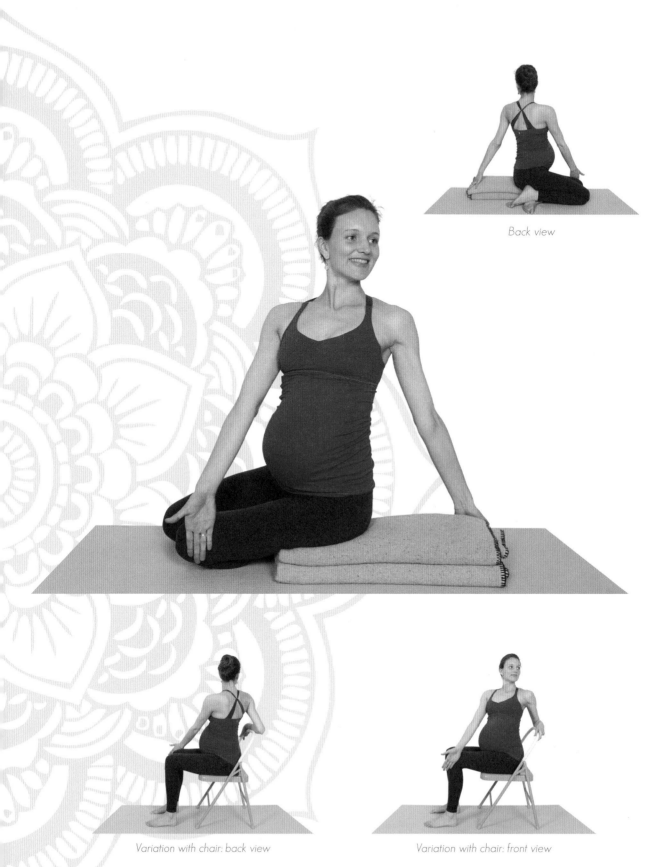

Back view

Variation with chair: back view

Variation with chair: front view

Bharadvajasana

Bharadvaja's Pose

This is an open twist that does not compress the belly. It opens the spine to create space and release in the mid and upper back.

Getting into the pose

1. Start in Dandasana, sitting on two blankets in Basic Fold (p. 6). The thighs should be off of the blankets.
2. Shift so that just the left sitting bone is on the blankets.
3. Lean over to your left and take your legs over to the right side.
4. Place the left foot under the right foot; the left toes point away from your midline and the right foot rests on the left arch, right toes point straight back (*Back view*).
5. Press your right hip down so the hip bones are level and in the same plane.
6. Take your left hand back to the floor or blankets behind you.
7. Take the back of your right hand to the outside of your right thigh, palm facing out, away from your thigh.

Engaging actions

1. Rotate the upper arms out and draw the shoulders away from the ears.
2. Exhale; press the left hand down and press the back of the right hand to the thigh; press the head of the thigh bones down.
3. Inhale; lift and broaden the chest.
4. Exhale; keeping the chest lifted, revolve the belly and chest to the left, letting your head follow.
5. With each inhalation keep lifting the spine and chest up; with each exhalation revolve further to the left.
6. Soften your eyes, relax your face, and let the breath flow freely.

Stay for 5–10 breaths.

Coming out of the pose

Unwind and release the legs to return to Dandasana.

Repeat on the other side.

Variation: with chair

The chair variation of this pose is a wonderful way to release back tension while sitting at your desk. It is also useful if you experience strain when your knees are folded, as in the classic pose. Refer to the Variation with chair: back view on opposite page.

1. Sit in a chair with your feet hip width apart, midline of the feet pointing straight forward.
2. Take your right hand to the backrest of the chair and the back of your left hand to the outer right thigh.
3. Rotate the upper arms out and draw the shoulders away from your ears.
4. Exhale; press the feet and sit bones down.
5. Inhale; lift and broaden the chest fully.
6. Keeping the chest lifted, on your next exhalation rotate the belly and chest; let your head follow.
7. Soften your eyes, relax your tongue, and let the breath flow freely.

Stay for 5-10 breaths

Coming Out of the Pose

Release the right hand and return to facing straight forward.

Repeat on the other side.

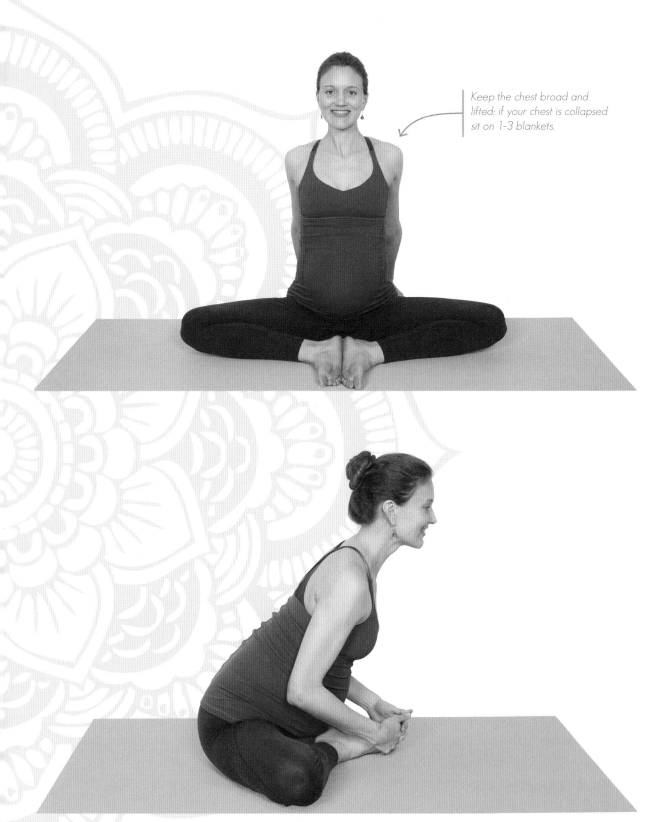

Keep the chest broad and lifted; if your chest is collapsed sit on 1-3 blankets.

Variation: Forward fold

Baddha Konasana
Bound Angle Pose

This is one of the best poses to practice while pregnant. It opens the hips, eases common prenatal discomforts, and prepares the body for labor.

NOTE

If baby is not head down at the end of pregnancy (after about 34 weeks), discontinue this pose.

You can also practice this pose with your back against the wall for more stability and ease.

GETTING INTO THE POSE

1. Start in Dandasana, sitting on one to three basic folded blankets.
2. Take your right hand to your inner right knee; use your hand to bend and slide your knee out to the right side; do the same action on the left side.
3. Bring the soles of your feet together.
4. Draw the feet as close as you can in toward the perineum.
5. Bring your fingertips to the floor or blankets behind you.

ENGAGING ACTIONS

1. From the inner knees, press the heels together.
2. From the inner groins extend out through the inner knees.
3. From the outer knees draw the outer thighs into your hips and plug the hips in.
4. Draw the skin of the buttock down toward the floor.
5. Exhale; press the hands down and press the outer knees down toward the floor.
6. Inhale; lift and broaden the chest.
7. Soften your eyes, relax your face, and let the breath flow freely.

Stay for 10–15 breaths.

COMING OUT OF THE POSE

1. Take your hands under the outer knees and lift the knees up.
2. Straighten the legs and return to Dandasana.

VARIATION: FORWARD FOLD

This is appropriate if you'd like more stretch and don't have low back, tailbone, or sacroiliac discomfort, and if your belly still has plenty of room as you come into the forward fold.

1. From Baddha Konasana, bring your hands to the floor in front of you.
2. Rotate the upper thighs from inner to outer.
3. Draw the skin of the buttock down toward the floor.
4. Lift and broaden the chest.
5. Keep the chest moving away from your navel as you fold forward from your hips; make sure there is plenty of space for baby.
6. From the inner knees, press the heels together.
7. From the inner groins extend out through the inner knees.
8. From the outer knees draw the outer thighs into your hips and plug the hips in.
9. Keep drawing the sternum bone away from the navel.

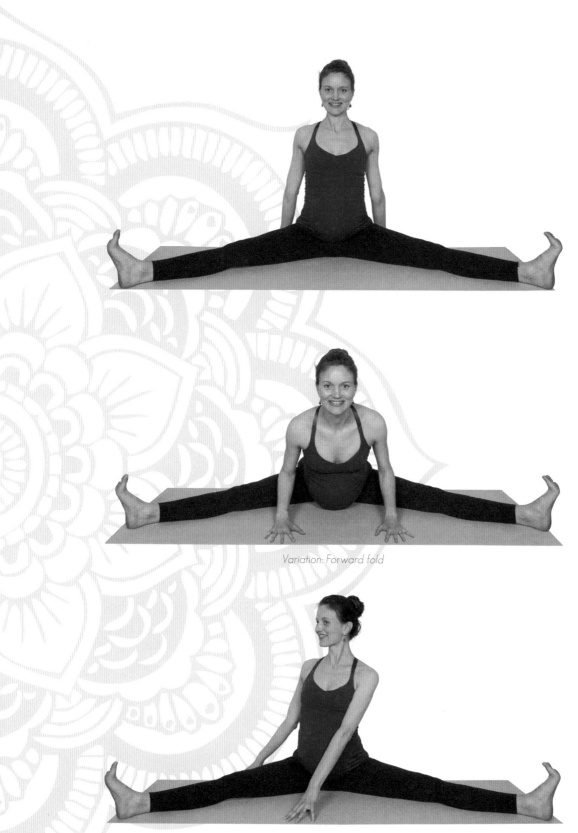

Variation: Forward fold

Variation: Twist

Upavista Konasana
Seated Wide Angle Pose

Like Baddha Konasana (previous page), this is one of the best poses to practice during pregnancy and in preparation for labor. Incorporating both of these poses into a daily practice will yield great benefits.

Note

If you are able to sit on the floor with the spine perfectly vertical, then you can do this pose without a blanket. If it is hard to keep the chest lifted, sit on one to two basic folded blankets.

Discontinue this pose toward the end of pregnancy (after about 34 weeks) if baby is not head down.

Getting into the Pose

1. Sit in Dandasana.
2. Take the legs wide apart.
3. Place the hands by your sides.
4. The spine should be vertical; if you find your upper back rounding, sit up on basic folded blankets as needed.
5. Point the big toes and the center of the knees straight up.

Engaging Actions

1. Extend strongly out through the inner heels and big toe mounds.
2. Exhale; press the hands down; press the top of the thighs firmly down.
3. Inhale; lift and broaden the chest; lift the sternum bone higher and higher.
4. Soften your eyes, relax your face, and let the breath flow freely

Stay for up to 10–15 breaths.

Coming Out of the Pose

Take your legs together and return to Dandansa.

Variation: Forward Fold

This is appropriate if you'd like more stretch and don't have low back, tailbone, or sacroiliac discomfort. Be sure you only fold forward as far as you can without putting any pressure on the belly.

1. Come to Upavista Konasana. Move the skin of the buttock down toward the floor.
2. Bring your hands to the floor in front of you.
3. Keeping the upper thighs rotating back and down and the chest lifted, fold forward from your hips; make sure there is plenty of space for baby.
4. Exhale; keep pressing the tops of the thighs down.
5. Inhale; draw the sternum bone away from the navel.
6. Soften your eyes, relax your face, and let the breath flow freely.

Variation: Twist

This variation creates length and openness in the spine.

1. From Upavista Konasana, take your right hand behind you.
2. Take your left hand in front of you on the floor.
3. Rotate the upper arms out and draw the shoulders away from the ears.
4. Exhale; press the hands down and press the head of the thigh bones down.
5. Inhale; lift and broaden the chest.
6. Keeping the chest lifted, exhale; revolve the belly and chest to the right, letting your head follow.
7. With each inhalation, keep lifting the chest up more; with each exhalation, revolve further to the right.

Release and repeat on the other side.

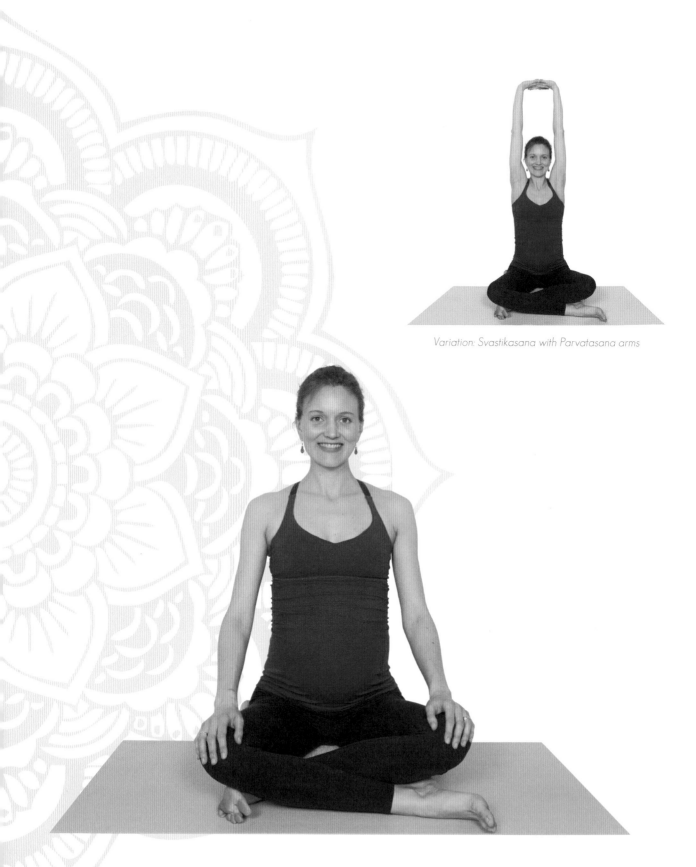

Variation: Svastikasana with Parvatasana arms

Svastikasana
Cross Legged Pose

This is a basic seated posture. It helps strengthen the muscles around the spine, open the hips, and prepare for labor.

Getting into the pose

1. Start in Dandasana, sitting on one to three basic folded blankets; have enough blankets so that your knees are in line with or lower than your hips when you are in the full pose.
2. Bend your left knee and place the right foot under the left knee; the shinbone should be more or less parallel with your torso.
3. Do the same with the right leg and foot, placing the right shin in front of the left.
4. Place your hands on your thighs.
5. Balance the weight equally on your sitting bones, spread the weight evenly from left to right and also from front to back.

Engaging actions

1. Draw the shoulders back and down.
2. Exhale; press the sitting bones down.
3. Inhale; lift and broaden the chest.
4. Soften your eyes, relax your face, and let the breath flow freely.

Stay for a few breaths or as long as a few minutes.

Change the cross of the legs and repeat on the other side. Return to Dandasana.

Variation: Svastikasana with Parvatasana arms

This variation opens the chest and strengthens the arms and back muscles. It is uplifting to the spirit.

1. Sit in Svastikasana.
2. Extend your arms out in front of you, parallel with the floor.
3. Interlace your hands all the way up to the webbing of your fingers and turn your palms away from you.
4. Lift your arms up over your head.
5. Extend the mound of the pointer fingers up and draw the little fingers back and down toward your head; the arms should be parallel to each other and in line with the ears.
6. Exhale; draw the shoulders back and down; press the sitting bones down.
7. Inhale; lift and broaden the chest.

Coming out of the pose

Release your hands down by your sides and repeat with the opposite pointer finger interlaced on top.

Return to Dandasana.

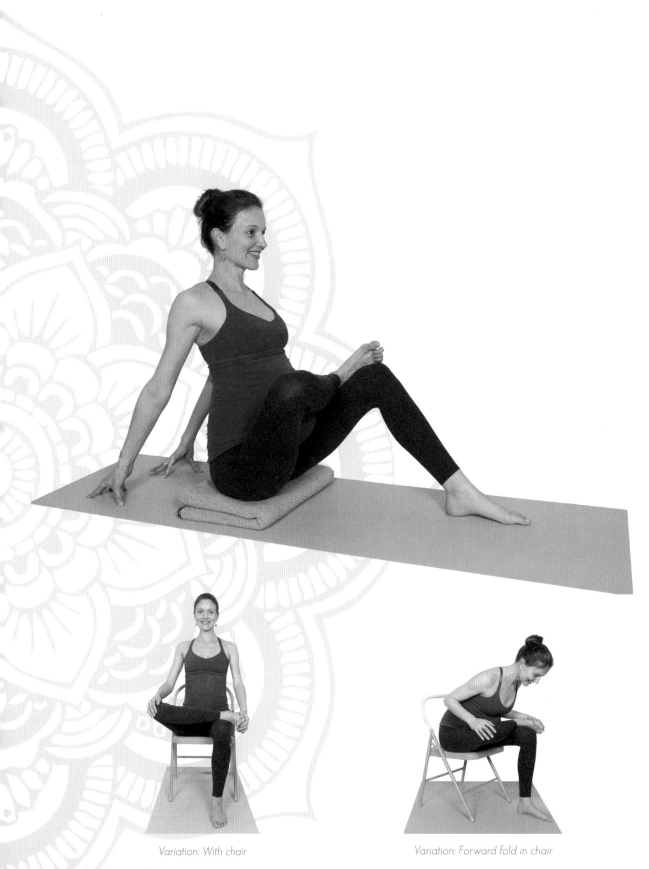

Variation: With chair

Variation: Forward fold in chair

Seated Window Stretch

This simple pose is a wonderful hip opener, which is a great pose for birth preparation and releasing tight hips and back tension.

Getting into the pose

1. Start in Dandasana, sitting on two to three blankets in Basic Fold (p. 6).
2. Bend the knees and place your feet flat on the floor.
3. Place your hands on the floor and lean back slightly.
4. Place your right ankle on your left thigh, just below the knee.

Engaging actions

1. Rotate the upper arms out and move the shoulders away from your ears.
2. Exhale; press your hands down; press firmly out through the right inner heel and big toe mound to flex the foot.
3. Inhale; lift and broaden the chest.
4. Soften your eyes, relax your face, and let the breath flow freely.

Stay for 5–10 breaths.

Note

To deepen the stretch you can press the right knee farther away from your torso and walk the left foot closer to your body (if your belly still has plenty of space).

To come out of the pose

Release the right leg and return to Dandasana.

Repeat on the other side.

Variation: With chair

You can do this same pose sitting in a chair. This variation is easier in later stages of pregnancy when the belly has grown bigger. This is a great way to relieve hip and low back tension while sitting at your desk, or anywhere. Be sure to keep the left foot pointing straight forward with the knee in line with the ankle.

Variation: Forward fold in chair

This is appropriate if you'd like more stretch and don't have low back, tailbone, or sacroiliac discomfort.

1. Keeping the chest lifted, fold forward from your hips, making sure there is plenty of space for baby.
2. Exhale; press firmly out through the right inner heel and big toe mound to flex the foot; press the left foot firmly to the floor.
3. Inhale; draw the sternum bone away from the navel.
4. Release and repeat on the other side.

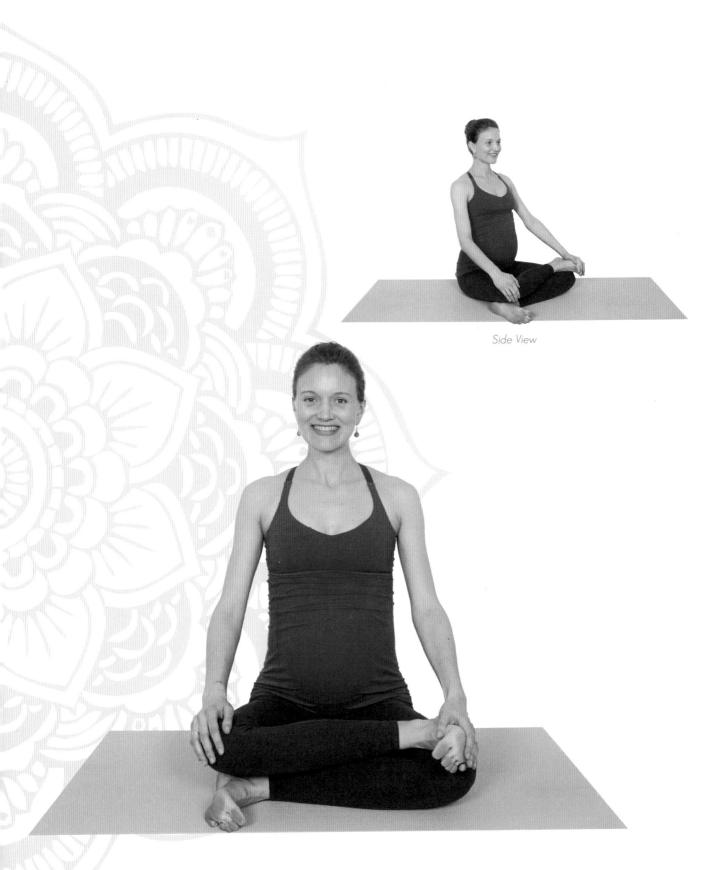

Side View

Agni Stambhasana
Burning Logs Pose

This pose opens the hips deeply.

Getting into the pose

1. Start in Dandasana, sitting on one to three blankets in Basic Fold (p. 6).
2. Take your left hand to your inner left knee and bend and slide your knee out to the left side.
3. Place your left ankle under your right knee.
4. Take your right hand to your inner right knee and bend and slide your knee out to the right side.
5. Place the right ankle just behind the left knee on the thigh; the shinbones should be close to in line with each other.
6. Rest your hands on your thighs or the floor.

Engaging actions

1. Press out firmly through both inner heels and big toe mounds to flex the feet.
2. Exhale; press your sitting bones evenly down.
3. Inhale; lift and broaden the chest.
4. Soften your eyes, relax your face, and let the breath flow freely.

Stay for 5–10 breaths.

Note

If your top knee is way up in the air away from your lower leg then try sitting on more blankets in Basic Fold.

Coming out of the pose

1. With your right hand, take hold of the right ankle and take your foot to the floor.
2. Straighten the legs and return to Dandasana.

Repeat on the other side.

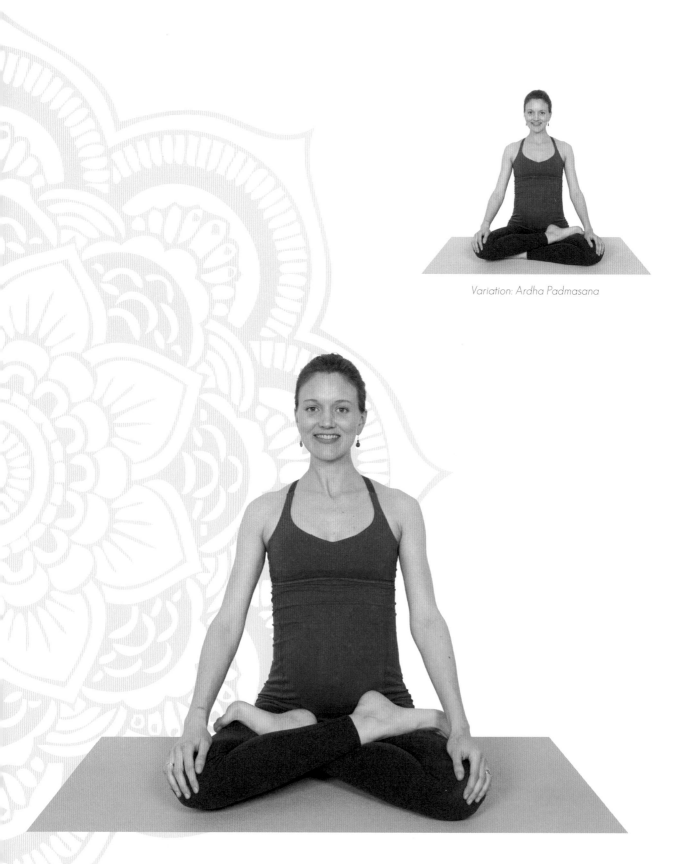

Variation: Ardha Padmasana

Padmasana

Lotus Pose

This is a classic yoga pose that is a deep hip opener. It is a traditional posture for practicing pranayama and meditation.

NOTE

This pose is not one to begin when pregnant; it is for practitioners who have already been practicing it prior to pregnancy. If this pose does not feel good in your knees, back, or hips then discontinue and practice Svastikasana (p. 97) instead. Also be mindful so that the heels do not press into the belly.

GETTING INTO THE POSE

1. Sit in Dandasana.
2. Take your right hand to your inner right knee and bend and slide your knee out to the right side.
3. Take hold of the outer ankle, and place the right foot high up on the left thigh near the groin.
4. Take your left hand to your inner left knee and bend and slide your knee out to the left side.
5. Take your hands under the left ankle and place the left foot high up on the left thigh near the groin; be sure that the heels don't compress the belly.
6. Place the hands on the floor or on the legs.

ENGAGING ACTIONS

1. Exhale; press your sitting bones evenly down; press the shinbones down.
2. Inhale; lift and broaden the chest; lift the waist and side body up.
3. Draw the knees closer together so the spine can lift more.
4. Soften your eyes, relax your face, and let the breath flow freely.

Stay for 5–10 breaths.

COMING OUT OF THE POSE

Release the legs and return to Dandasana.

Repeat on the other side.

VARIATION: ARDHA PADMASANA

Like full Lotus Pose, this should only be practiced if you were already doing it prior to becoming pregnant. It is the same as Padmasana except that the left foot rests on the floor, under the right shin, instead of on the right thigh.

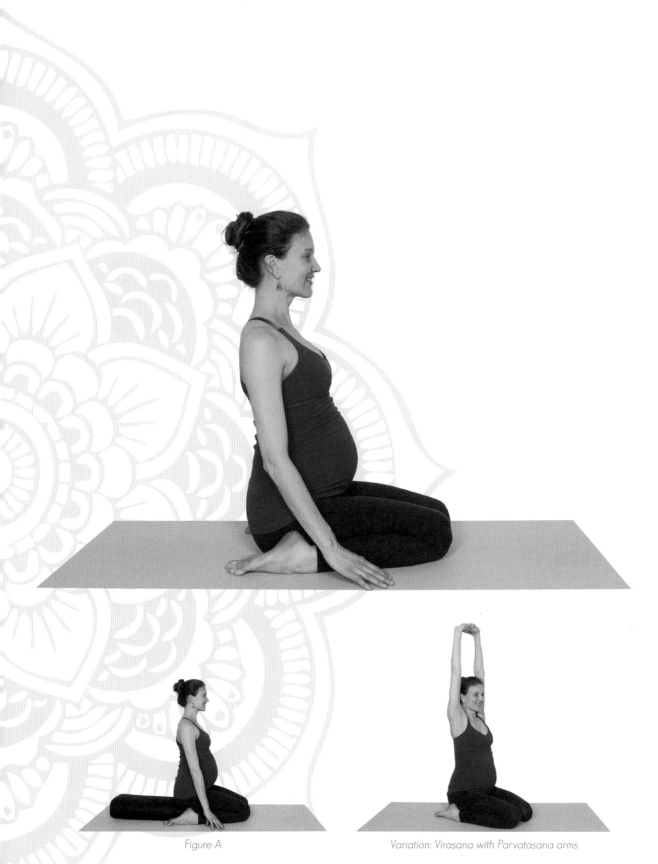

Figure A

Variation: Virasana with Parvatasana arms

Virasana
Hero's Pose

This is a grounding pose that can help prevent varicose veins and edema.

NOTE

If you feel pressure in your knees or ankles in this pose, then sit on more height (*Figure A*).

GETTING INTO THE POSE

1. Place a bolster or a couple of blankets in Narrow Fold (p. 6) at the back of your sticky mat; have the shorter side of the props pointing forward. If you can sit comfortably on the floor without prop support then do so.
2. Kneel in front of the props, facing away from them; have the feet on either side of the narrow aspect of the bolster/blankets and the big toes pointing straight back.
3. Take hold of the calves right behind the knees and roll the flesh of the calves out away from the midline and back toward the feet.
4. Sit down on the bolster/blankets; make sure only the sitting bones are on the props, not the thighs.
5. Roll the calves out to the sides away from the midline and draw the outer ankles in.
6. Spread your toes and press the little toes to the floor with your hands.

ENGAGING ACTIONS

1. Exhale; draw the shoulders back and down; press the sitting bones down; keep pressing the toes down.
2. Inhale; lift and broaden the chest.
3. Soften your eyes, relax your face, and let the breath flow freely.

DETAILS TO BE MINDFUL OF

Keep the thighs together. In later stages of pregnancy if the belly makes this impossible then bring the thighs apart as needed.

Stay for 5–10 breaths.

TO COME OUT OF THE POSE

1. Place the hands on the floor and come to hands and knees.
2. Stretch the legs out one at a time to open the backs of the knees.
3. Return to Dandasana.

VARIATION: VIRASANA WITH PARVATASANA ARMS

This variation opens the chest, strengthens the arms, and is uplifting to the spirit.

1. Sit in Virasana.
2. Extend your arms out in front of you, parallel with the floor.
3. Interlace your hands all the way up to the webbing of your fingers and turn your palms away from you.
4. Lift your arms up over your head.
5. Extend the mound of the pointer fingers up and draw the little fingers back and down toward your head; the arms should be parallel to each other and in line with the ears.
6. Exhale; press the sitting bones down; press the shinbones down; press the toes down.
7. Inhale; lift and broaden the chest and extend mounds of the pointer fingers up.
8. Relax the eyes, soften the tongue, and let the breath flow freely.

NOTE

You can also practice this pose with Gomukasana arms (p. 21).

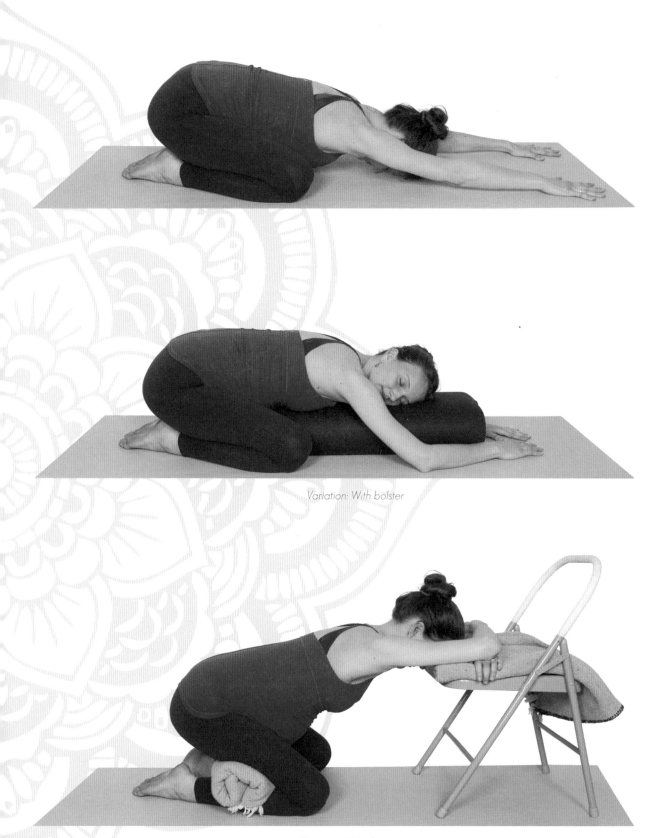

Variation: With bolster

Variation: With chair

Adho Mukha Virasana
Downward Facing Hero's Pose / Child's Pose

This is a fantastic pose to practice throughout pregnancy. It brings space to the spine and ribs and is a calming, quieting pose that is great to use as a resting point between more vigorous poses. With a stack of pillows under the chest, this is a wonderful pose for laboring during birth.

Note

This pose helps baby find a good position for birth. The baby's spine is heaviest, so when you are facing the floor, as in this pose, baby's spine is encouraged to rotate toward the floor. This positioning is optimal for birthing.

If your sitting bones don't easily reach your heels, put some narrow folded blankets between your sitting bones and calves.

Getting into the pose

1. Start on your hands and knees.
2. Take the knees wide (about as wide as your sticky mat).
3. Bring the big toes together and lower the sitting bones to the heels.
4. Extend the chest away from the belly to open the front of the body; maintain the extension of the front body as you take the forehead to the floor. Stretch the arms out beyond the head and extend them fully.

Engaging actions

1. Inhale; breathe space into your lower back.
2. Exhale; draw the sitting bones toward the heels and relax your head and arms fully.
3. Soften your eyes, relax your face, and let the breath flow freely.

Stay for up to 5-10 minutes.

Variation: with bolster

This variation is great as pregnancy advances and the belly needs more space. Take a bolster under the chest and rest the side of your head on it. You want the pose to be restful and the belly to have plenty of room so it doesn't feel compressed.

Variation: with chair

If you have heartburn, practicing this pose upright with a chair can be more comfortable. Lay a blanket over the chair to cushion your head. You can also try putting a rolled blanket between the thighs and calves for extra comfort and support.

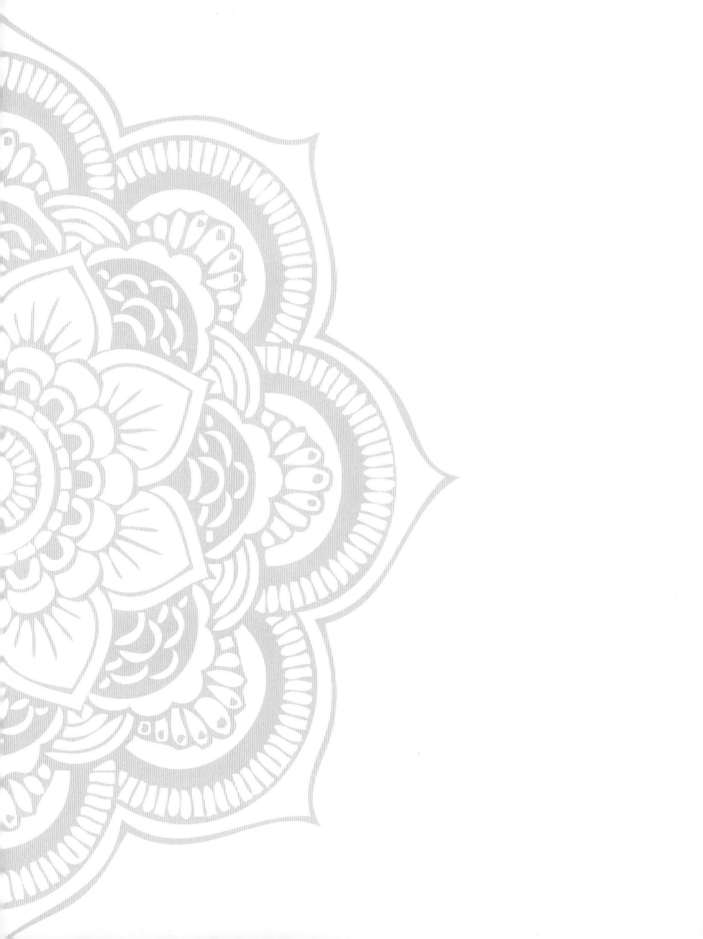

INVERSIONS

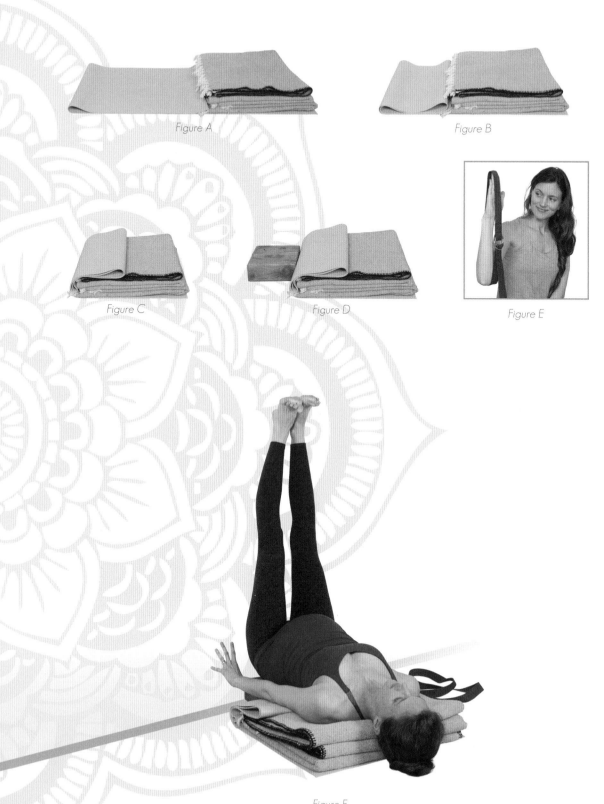

Figure A

Figure B

Figure C

Figure D

Figure E

Figure F

Salamba Sarvangasana
Shoulder Stand

This pose is known as the "Queen" of all poses due to its importance in restoring vitality. It is a fantastic pose for calming the mind and supporting the nervous system, cardiovascular system, immune system, and reproductive system. It also relieves gastric issues like constipation and flatulence, both of which are more common during pregnancy.

NOTE

This pose is not one to begin during pregnancy. If you have never practiced this pose before, skip this pose and instead do Chatushpadasana (p. 125), Setu Bandha Sarvangasana (p. 141) or Viparita Karani (p. 147). If you had a confident Shoulder Stand practice prior to pregnancy, it is still recommended that you have someone spot you in the pose.

GETTING INTO THE POSE

1. Stack 3 blankets in Open Fold (p. 6) on top of each other with the smooth edge of the blankets to the edge of the sticky mat and each blanket staggered slightly inward (*Figure A*).
2. Fold the other end of the sticky mat up against the edge of the blankets (*Figure B*) and then fold the edge one more time (*Figure C*).
3. Place two blocks lengthwise against the wall and have the sticky mat set up right against the blocks (*Figure D*).
4. Make a loop in the belt that is the same length as the distance from elbow to extended middle finger (*Figure E*).
5. Lie down on the props so the sacrum, neck, and shoulders are supported by the blankets and blocks. The head is off of the blankets; look straight up toward the ceiling and hold the belt loop in your right hand (*Figure F*).

6. Extend the legs straight up the wall. Press the hands to the floor, and keeping the heels where they are on the wall take the toes to the wall to lift the hips up.
7. Bend the knees and lift the hips higher; under your back, place the loop of the belt over your arms and just above the elbows.
8. Straighten the arms so the fingers point to the wall.
9. Rotate the upper arms strongly out away from your midline to come onto the outer shoulders; this action is very important for your neck.
10. Bend your elbows and place your hands on your back; walk your hands down your back as much as you can and lift the hips higher.
11. Press the outer elbows and outer shoulders down and lift the sitting bones to the backs of the knees; from the back of the knees draw the hamstring to the buttock and firm the thighs (*Figure G*); stay here if this is as far as you'd like to go.
12. If you'd like to go further, keep the legs firm and extend the right foot straight up to the ceiling; extend firmly through the inner heel and big toe mound and straighten the leg fully (*Figure H*).
13. Take a few breaths; return the right foot to the wall and do the same with the left foot.
14. If you are feeling very stable then extend the right leg away from the wall, too (*Figure I*).

continued on next page

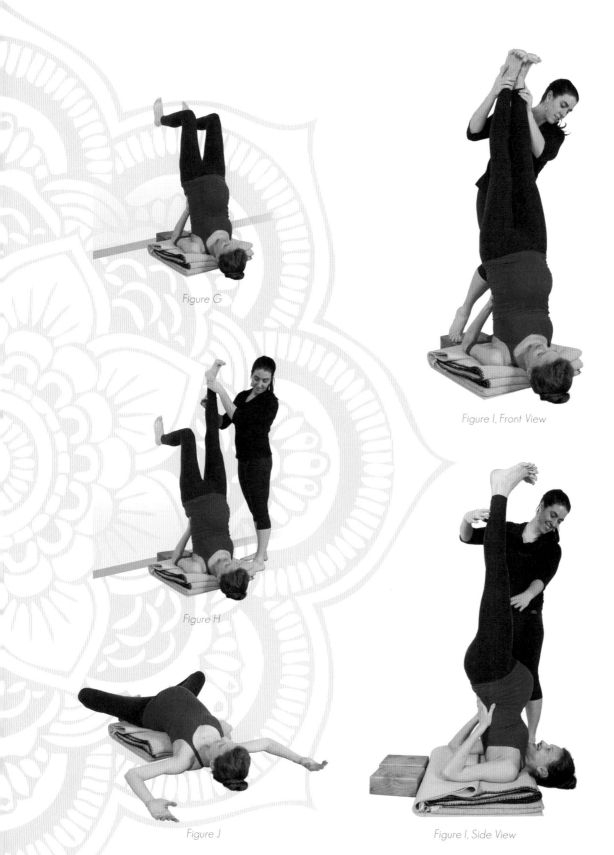

Figure G

Figure H

Figure J

Figure I, Front View

Figure I, Side View

Engaging actions

1. Take the inner ankles together; extend strongly up through the inner heels and big toe mounds.
2. Rotate the front of the thighs in, broadening the backs of the thighs.
3. Draw the tailbone in and the sitting bones to the backs of the knees.
4. Press the inner thighs back.
5. Exhale; press the outer elbows down.
6. Inhale; extend strongly up through the inner heels and big toe mounds.
7. Soften your eyes, relax your face, and let the breath flow freely.

Details to be mindful of

- Be sure that there is no compression in the neck or throat.
- The breath should be able to flow freely while in the pose; if it is difficult to breathe then come down.

Stay for 5-10 breaths.

Getting out of the pose

1. Take the feet back to the wall one by one. Remove the belt and lower down one by one vertebrae until the back is resting on the blankets.
2. Press your feet to the wall and slide off the blankets so the tips of the shoulder blades come just off the blankets.
3. Relax your legs into Baddha Konasana and rest the arms in line with the shoulders (*Figure J*).
4. Rest here for a few breaths and then bend the knees and roll over to your side and come up.

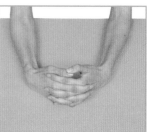

Figure B

It is crucial to keep the inner shoulder blades lifted to keep the neck protected and safe; come down right away if the shoulder blades are not staying lifted.

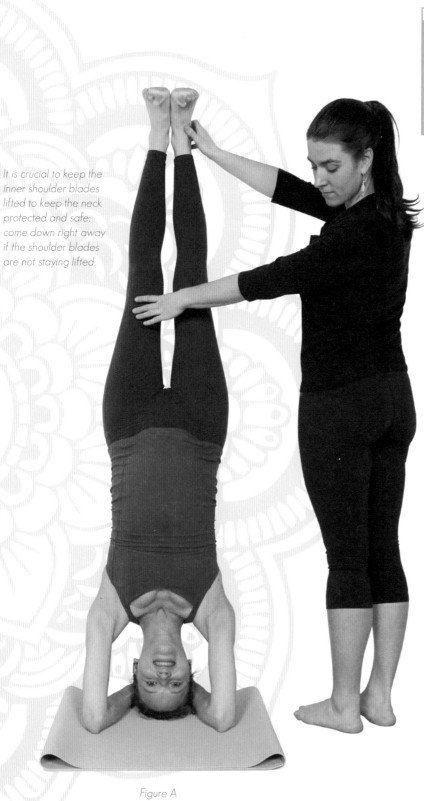

Figure A

Salamba Sirsasana
Supported Head Balance Pose

This pose is known as the "King" of all poses; it deeply restores all of the body systems. It is revitalizing and uplifting and can help relieve leg cramps. Being upside down is a great way to reset your energy and attitude.

Note

This pose is not one to begin during pregnancy. If you had a confident Head Stand practice prior to pregnancy, you may continue this pose with the spotting assistance of a skilled teacher.

When you practice Sirsasana it is important to do Sarvangasana in the same practice, at some point after Sirsasana and for at least the same duration. Practicing Sirsasana without Sarvangasana is known to create agitation and irritation.

For more advanced stages of pregnancy, have the feet hip width apart to accommodate the baby. In the second trimester, try having the heels apart; in the third trimester, try having the feet apart.

Getting into the pose

1. Fold your sticky mat into thirds.
2. Start on your hands and knees.
3. Interlace your hands all the way up to the webbing of the fingers.
4. Place your knuckles against the wall, elbows shoulder width apart.
5. Place your head deep in your hands and place the crown of the head on the floor.
6. Place one thumb over the other (*Figure B*).
7. Press the bottom wrists firmly down to the floor and press the top wrists into your head.
8. Lift the shoulders away from your ears.
9. Press the inner elbows down, turn the toes under, and lift the hips up like in Adho Mukha Svanasana (p. 69).
10. Keep lifting the shoulders up, away from the head.
11. Extend one leg up toward the ceiling like in Eka Pada Adho Mukha Svanasana (p. 73), and rotate the lifted hip down to make the hips level; take the opposite hip toward the center of the room.
12. Bend the knee of the foot that is on the floor. Give a little kick and bring the lifted leg up to the wall.

Engaging actions

1. Bring the inner ankles together and rotate the front of the thighs in to broaden the low back.
2. Take the tailbone in and move the sitting bones to the heels.
3. Extend strongly up through the inner heels and the big toe mounds; firm the thighs and straighten the legs fully.
4. Exhale; press the forearms and the crown of the head down.
5. Inhale; lift the inner shoulder blades up and draw them into the spine; keep extending out through the inner heels and big toe mounds.
6. Soften your eyes, relax your face, and let the breath flow freely.

Details to be mindful of

- To keep from overarching the back, draw the front ribs into the back body.
- Never practice this pose if you feel strain in the neck; if it begins in the pose then come down immediately.

Stay for as long as you feel stable and can keep the shoulders lifted and the breath even and steady.

To come out of the pose

1. Press the forearms down and keep lifting the shoulders up as you lower first one leg and then the other.
2. Rest in Adho Mukha Virasana (p. 107).

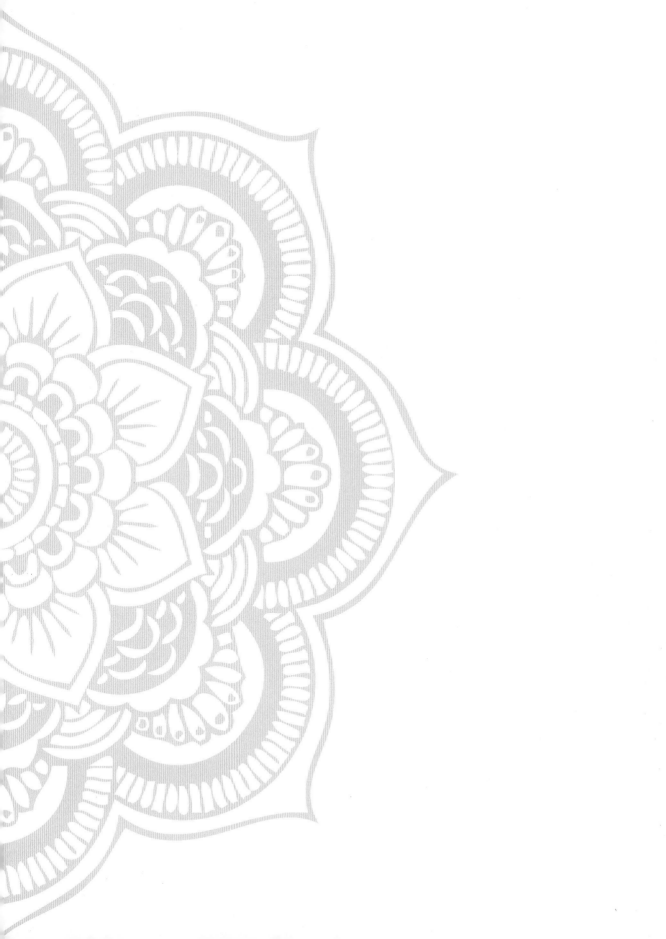

BACK BENDS

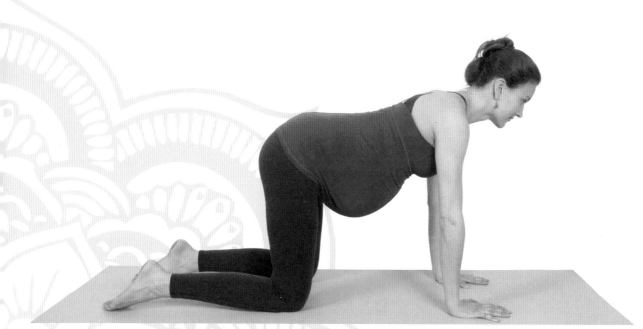

Figure A: Hands and Knees

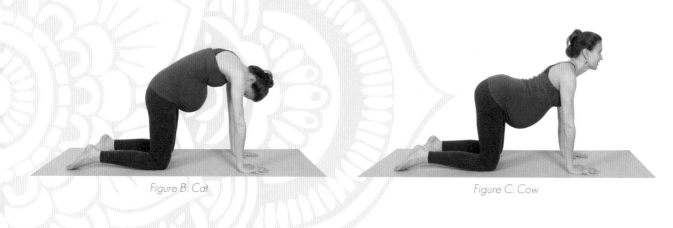

Figure B: Cat

Figure C: Cow

Draw the belly to the spine to avoid overarching the low back.

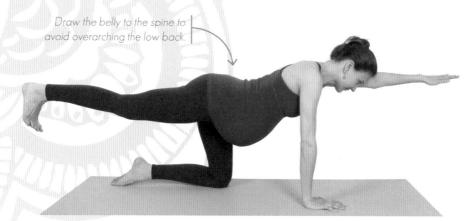

Figure D: Sundog

Cat • Cow • Sundog

These poses are a gentle yet effective way to warm up the spine with dynamic action. Starting with them is a great way to check in and notice how your back is feeling as you begin your practice, gently releasing tension and bringing awareness to sensitive and/or tight areas.

NOTE

You can place an Open Open Fold blanket (p. 7) on your sticky mat to make these poses more comfortable for your knees.

CAT • COW

1. Start on your hands and knees; have your wrists in line with your shoulders and your knees in line with your hips (*Figure A: Hands and Knees*).
2. Spread the fingers wide and press the mounds of the fingers firmly down.
3. Rotate the upper arms out to broaden and open the chest and draw the shoulders away from the ears.
4. Draw the chest away from the belly.
5. Take a deep breath in and arch the upper back; taking your sternum bone further away from your navel, look up.
6. Exhale; round the spine beginning with the tailbone then low back, mid back, upper back, and head (*Figure B: Cat*).
7. Inhale; arch the spine one vertebrae at a time, beginning with the tailbone and ending with the chest and head (*Figure C: Cow*).
8. Soften your eyes, relax your face, and let the breath flow freely.

Continue alternating between the two variations, following the breath, for 5–10 breaths.

When you are finished, rest in Adho Mukha Virasana (p. 107).

SUNDOG

1. From hands and knees, rotate the upper arms out away from the midline and take the shoulders away from your ears.
2. Draw the sternum bone away from the navel and take the belly toward the spine (*Figure A: Hands and Knees*).
3. Inhale; extend the left arm up in line with the left ear and reach strongly out through the fingertips.
4. Lift the right leg up so it is parallel with the floor; point the toes straight down toward the floor.
5. Extend firmly out through the right inner heel and big toe mound; straighten your arm and leg fully (*Figure D: Sundog*).
6. Exhale; come back to hands and knees.
7. Inhale; extend the right arm and left leg this time.
8. Repeat actions #4 through #7.

Continue alternating between sides, following the breath, for 5–10 breaths.

When you are finished rest in Adho Mukha Virasana (p. 107).

NOTE

For a more intense version of this pose, hold each side for 5–10 breaths. For a less intense version of this pose, try extending only the arm or only the leg each time.

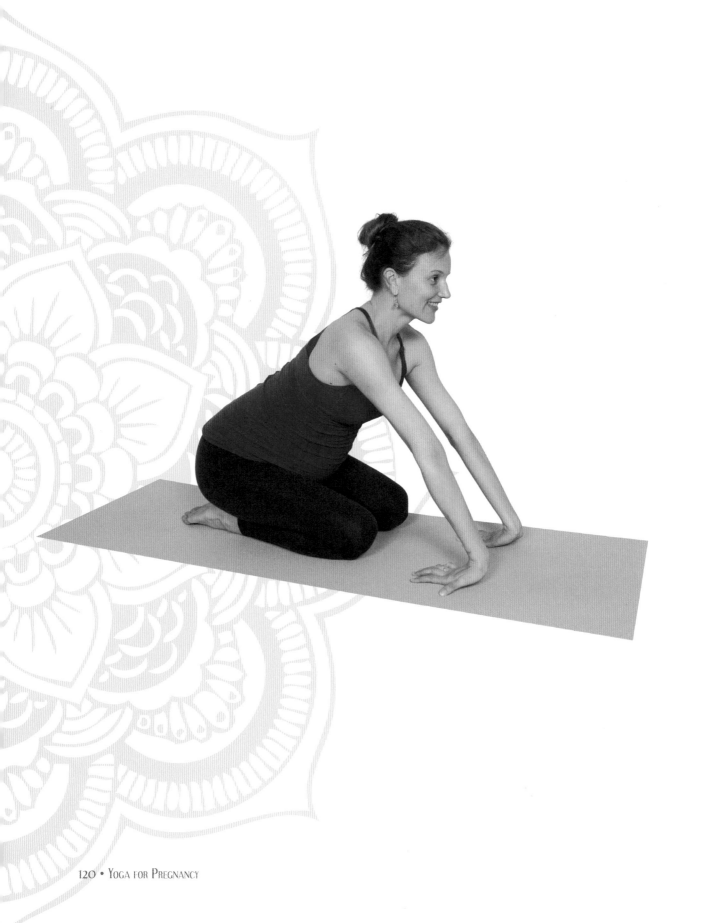

Wrist Stretch

This pose helps relieve wrist tension and pain by opening the carpal tunnels.

1. From hands and knees, turn the hands so the fingers point toward your knees, the thumbs pointing away from each other.
2. Draw the shoulders away from the ears and move the chest away from the belly.
3. If this is plenty of stretch, stay here; to deepen the stretch, gradually take the sitting bones back toward the heels.

Stay for 5–10 breaths.

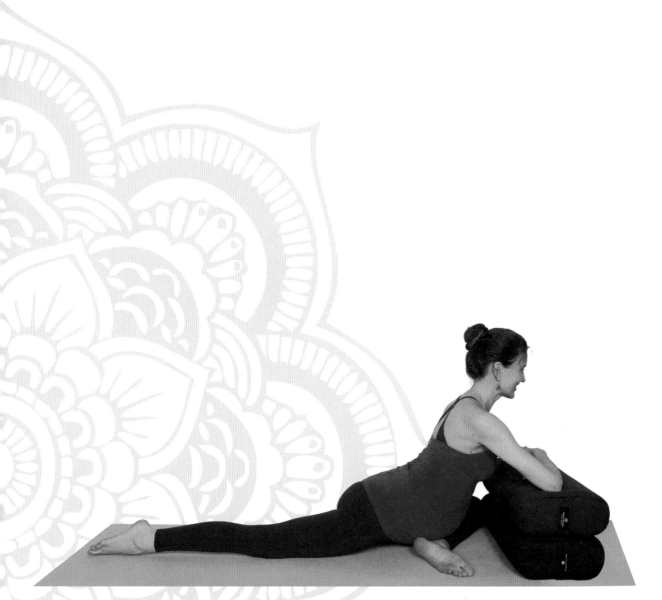

Eka Pada Rajakapotanasana
One Legged King Pigeon Pose

This poses opens the hips, helping to prepare for labor.

NOTE

The variation shown here is the first stage of the pose and uses props to help make it comfortable and safe during pregnancy. If you'd like extra padding, lay a blanket in Open Open Fold (p. 7) on top of your sticky mat.

GETTING INTO THE POSE

1. Begin on your hands and knees.
2. Take the left knee forward and away from the midline so there is plenty of space for your belly.
3. Bring the left foot forward, away from your body.
4. Extend the right leg straight back; point and reach through the inner right big toe.
5. Place your hands on the floor in front of you or rest your forearms on a bolster or two (find the right height so that your belly has plenty of room and is not compressed in any way).

ENGAGING ACTIONS

1. Rotate the front right hip bone toward the floor so your hips and both sides of your low back are level.
2. Take your tailbone in and the sitting bones toward the backs of the knees.
3. Exhale; draw the shoulders away from the ears.
4. Inhale; lift and broaden the chest; lift the lower belly up and lengthen the side body up.
5. Soften your eyes, relax your face, and let the breath flow freely.

Stay for 5–10 breaths.

TO COME OUT OF THE POSE

Press your hands to the floor; take the left leg back and return to hands and knees.

Repeat on the second side.

Note: For earlier stages of pregnancy and if you'd like more hip opening, you can lower your torso down toward the floor as long as there is still plenty of room for baby.

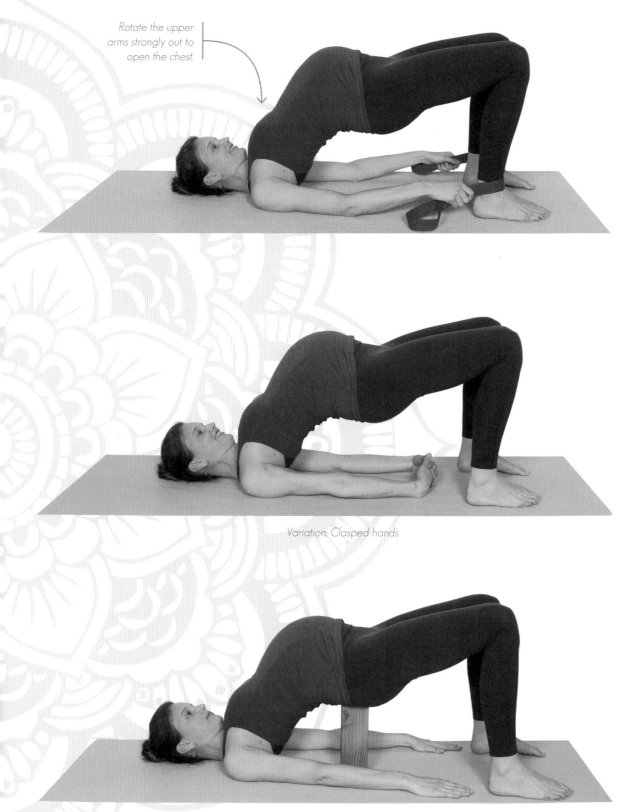

Rotate the upper arms strongly out to open the chest.

Variation: Clasped hands

Variation: With block

Chatushpadasana
Four Limb Pose

This pose opens the shoulders and chest and strengthens the legs. It teaches the shoulder action needed for Sarvagasana (Shoulder Stand Pose, p. 111).

NOTE

Avoid this pose in the first trimester and later in the third trimester. If the pose is not comfortable in later stages of pregnancy, discontinue.

GETTING INTO THE POSE

1. Lie on the floor on your back.
2. Place the feet on the floor and walk them in toward the buttock; have the feet hip width apart and the outer edges of the feet parallel.
3. Place a belt around the ankles.
4. Walk your hands down your belt as close to the feet as you can.
5. Take a deep breath in.
6. Exhale; press the inner heels firmly into the floor and lift the hips up.

ENGAGING ACTIONS

1. Rotate the upper arms strongly out to open the chest.
2. Take the tailbone in and the sitting bones toward the backs of the knees.
3. Rotate the thighs in so they are parallel to each other.
4. Exhale; from the backs of the knees draw the hamstring toward the buttock and lift the middle buttock up; lift the chest.
5. Soften your eyes, relax your face, and let the breath flow freely.

Stay for 5 breaths.

COMING OUT OF THE POSE

Roll down through the spine vertebrae by vertebrae, starting at the upper back and ending at the tailbone.

VARIATION: CLASPED HANDS

This variation supports the action of rolling the upper arms out, creating openness in the heart.

VARIATION: WITH BLOCK

Using a block under the sacrum provides extra support and stability.

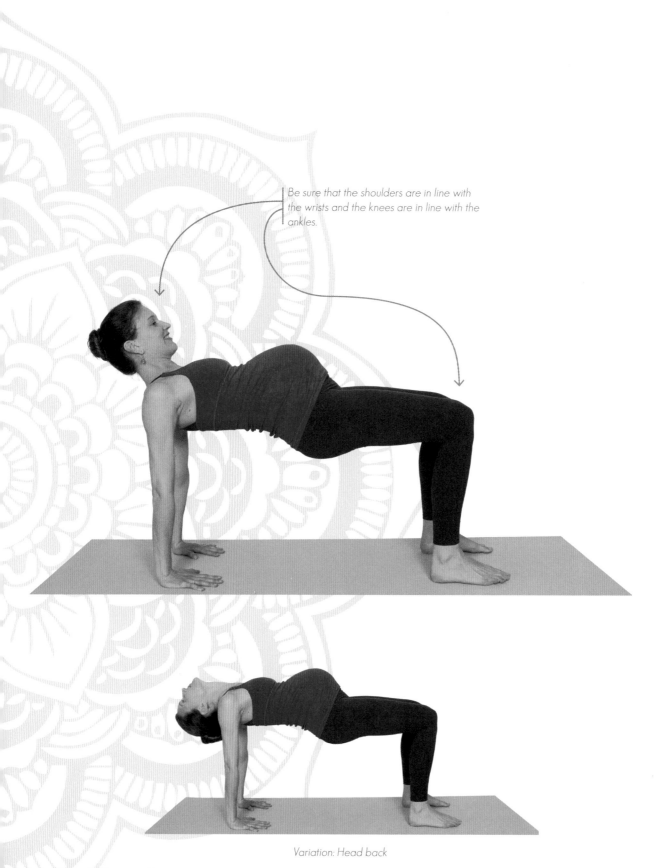

Be sure that the shoulders are in line with the wrists and the knees are in line with the ankles.

Variation: Head back

Purvottanasana
Intense Stretch of the East

This is one of few back bends that can be done during pregnancy, creating a sense of openness in the front body. The full version of this pose is not included in these instructions and is not recommended during pregnancy.

Getting into the pose

1. Sit in Dandasana.
2. Bend the knees and place the feet on the floor hip width apart, outer edges of the feet parallel.
3. Place the palms a few inches behind you, shoulder width apart.
4. Turn the fingers toward you and rotate the upper arms out away from your midline.
5. Press the hands and feet down to lift the hips up; straighten the arms.

Engaging actions

1. Move the sitting bones toward the backs of the knees.
2. From the back of the knees draw the hamstrings to the buttock.
3. Exhale; press the hands down; from the backs of the knees press the inner heels firmly down.
4. Inhale; lift the middle buttock higher; lift and open the chest; lift up and out of the shoulders.
5. Soften your eyes, relax your face, and let the breath flow freely.

Stay for 5–10 breaths.

Coming out of the pose

Lower back to the floor and straighten the legs to return to Dandasana.

Note

If you feel a significant stretch in your belly in this posture, back off or discontinue the pose all together. You do not want to feel a stretch in the abdominal area.

Variation: Head back

This variation opens the heart more fully and also opens and releases the muscles of the throat.

It is imperative to fully lift the chest before you take the head back so the neck is fully supported.

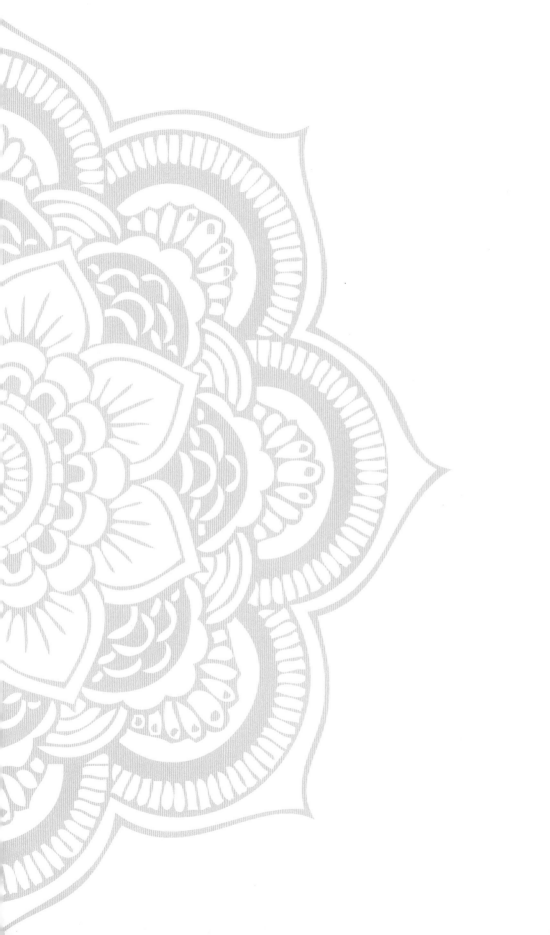

RESTORATIVES

Supta Padangustasana I

Roll the left thigh from inner to outer to keep the left side of torso long.

Supta Padangustasana I & II
Reclined Big Toe Pose

These are fabulous poses for opening the backs of the legs. They bring deep opening to the hamstring muscles while allowing the body to be in a restful position. In later stages of pregnancy, Supta Padangustasana I is no longer possible due to the size of the belly.

NOTE

When you get to the point in your pregnancy when you can no longer lie on your back, practice the supported variations of these poses.

GETTING INTO THE POSE

1. For Supta Padangustasana I, lie flat on the floor.
2. Bend the knees and place the feet on the floor hip width apart, outer edges of the feet parallel.
3. Take the left knee in toward your chest and place a belt around the pad of the left big toe mound; hold on to the two ends of the belt with each hand and straighten the left leg up to the ceiling.
4. Walk your hands as high up the belt as you can, keeping your arms and leg straight.
5. Rotate the upper arms out, taking the heads of the shoulders down to the floor to broaden and open the chest.
6. Rotate the left upper thigh away from your midline to lengthen the side body.
7. Straighten the right leg along the floor sharply, keeping the right kneecap and right big toe pointing straight up to the ceiling.

ENGAGING ACTIONS

1. Exhale; press your inner right thigh down.
2. Inhale; from the backs of the knees press firmly out through the inner heels and the big toe mounds; firm the kneecaps and straighten the legs fully.
3. Soften your eyes, relax your face, and let the breath flow freely.

Stay for 5–10 breaths.

COMING OUT OF THE POSE

1. Release the belt from your left foot.
2. Straighten your legs along the floor and notice the difference between the two sides.

Repeat on the second side.

continued on next page

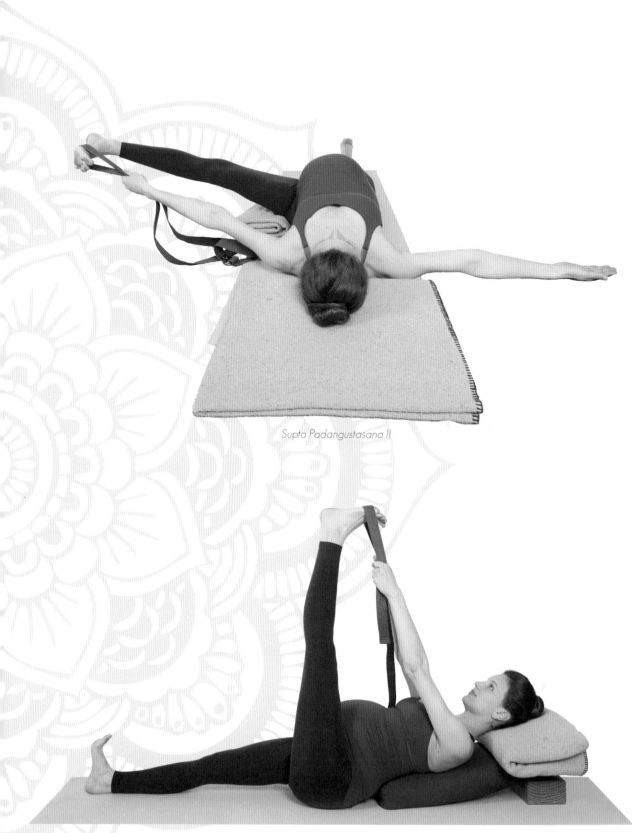

Supta Padangustasana II

Supported Supta Padangustasana I

SUPTA PADANGUSTASANA II

This next stage of the pose brings the stretch more deeply into the groin.

1. Place two Basic Fold blankets (p. 6) right next to your left outer hip. Follow the directions as in Supta Padangustasana I above and then, after step #2 in the engaging actions above, take the belt into the left hand only.

2. Be sure to keep rotating the left upper thigh out.

3. Lower your left leg toward the floor. Have your hip supported by the folded blankets.

4. Keep pressing the inner right thigh down.

5. Press strongly out through the inner heels and big toe mounds to straighten the legs fully.

SUPPORTED SUPTA PADANGUSTASANA I

This variation uses props to support you as the belly grows and it becomes uncomfortable to lie flat on your back. Once the belly reaches a certain size, Supta Padangustasana I is no longer possible.

1. Place a block toward the back of your sticky mat and lean a bolster against it; have the top of the bolster all the way supported by the block and the other end resting on the floor. Place a blanket at the higher end of the bolster, to be used as a pillow.

2. Before you lie back on the bolster be sure that there is a little space between your back and the bolster (enough so your fingers can fit between the two).

3. Proceed with Padangustasana I as described above. Be sure that the blanket used as a pillow is under the neck and head and the shoulders are not on the blanket.

SUPPORTED SUPTA PADANGUSTASANA II

(not shown)

Follow the same instructions for Supta Padangustasana II from above with the bolster and block set up described in Variation #2 Supported Supta Padangustasana I.

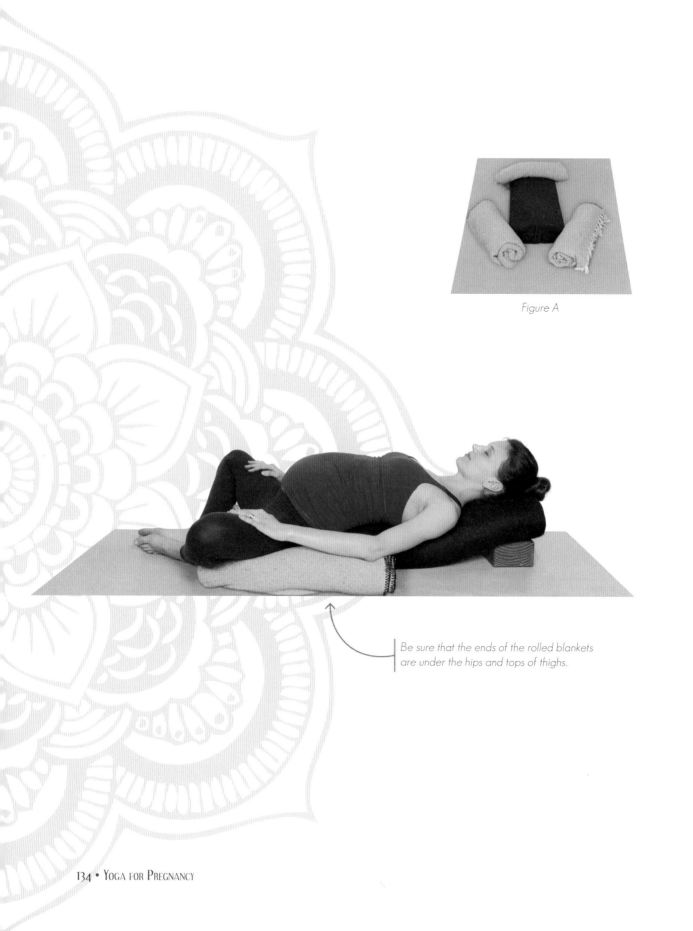

Figure A

Be sure that the ends of the rolled blankets
are under the hips and tops of thighs.

Supta Baddha Konasana
Reclined Bound Angle Pose

This is one of the best poses during pregnancy, bringing you back home to your center while opening the hips. It is a great pose to practice daily.

GETTING INTO THE POSE

1. Place a block at the back of your sticky mat and place one end of a bolster on the block; place two rolled blankets at an angle beside the bolster; if you like, place a blanket in Basic Fold at the top of the bolster for a pillow (*Figure A* and see pages 5–7 for prop descriptions).
2. Sit in Dandasana with your back a few inches away from the bolster.
3. Take your right hand to your inner right knee; use your hand to bend and slide your knee out to the right side; do the same action with your left leg.
4. Bring the soles of your feet together.
5. Draw the feet as close as you can in toward the perineum.
6. Place the rolled blankets under your upper thighs for support.
7. Lean back and lie down on the bolster.
8. If you're using a blanket under the head, adjust it so that it supports the whole head and neck, and just the shoulders are on the bolster.
9. Move the ends of the rolled blankets in toward your sides and rest your elbows on them.
10. Point the fingers up to the ceiling and press the elbows down to lift the chest up, drawing the shoulder blades into the back body (*Pranayama Figure A*, p. 155).
11. Keep the chest open and relax the hands down; the hands can be on the belly or inner thighs.

ENGAGING ACTIONS

1. Draw your shoulder blades down and away from your ears to open and broaden your chest.
2. Move your sit bones toward your heels to broaden and lengthen the low back.
3. Close your eyes and soften the entire surface of the face.
4. Let the eyes retreat deep into the skull.
5. Let the lower jaw release completely from the upper jaw.
6. Observe your breath and find quietness.

Stay for at least 5 minutes and for as long as you'd like.

COMING OUT OF THE POSE

1. Take the knees together, feet on the floor; then straighten the legs and lie still for a few breaths.
2. Bend the knees and roll over to your side; pause here for several breaths and then come up.

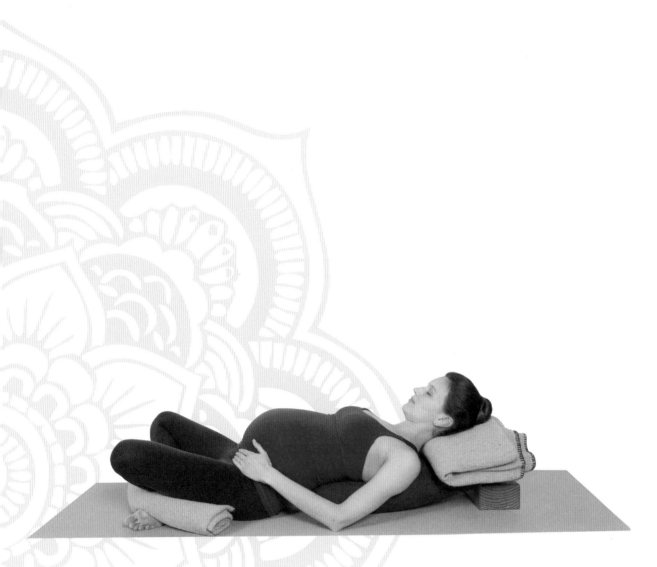

Supta Svastikasana
Reclined Cross-Legged Pose

This is a wonderful pose that opens the hips while you rest. It also eases heartburn and indigestion.

GETTING INTO THE POSE

1. Place a block at the back of your sticky mat and place one end of a bolster on the block.
2. Roll a blanket from half fold and have it near you; if you like, place a blanket in Basic Fold at the top of the bolster for a pillow.
3. Sit in Dandasana with your back a few inches away from the bolster.
4. Bend your right knee and place the right foot under the left knee; the shinbone should be more or less parallel with your torso.
5. Do the same with the left leg and foot, placing the left shin in front of the right.
6. Place your hands on your thighs.
7. Balance the weight equally on your sitting bones; spread the weight evenly from left to right and also from front to back.
8. Slide the rolled blanket under each of the shinbones.
9. Lift and broaden the chest; maintain the openness in the chest and lower the back onto the bolster.

ENGAGING ACTIONS

1. Draw the shoulders away from the ears and tuck the shoulder blades into the back to open the chest further.
2. Move your sitting bones toward your heels to broaden and lengthen the low back.
3. Close your eyes and soften the entire surface of the face.
4. Let the eyes retreat deep into the skull.
5. Let the lower jaw release completely from the upper jaw.
6. Observe your breath and find quietness.

Stay for at least a few minutes and for as long as you'd like.

COMING OUT OF THE POSE

1. Straighten the legs and lie still for a few breaths.
2. Bend the knees and roll over to your side; come up to sitting.

Change the cross of the legs and repeat.

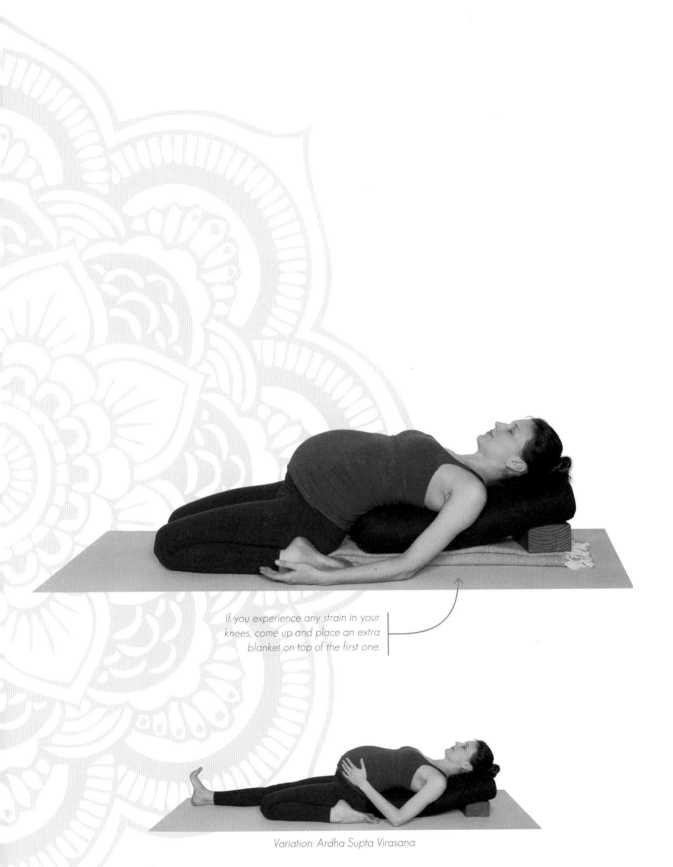

If you experience any strain in your knees, come up and place an extra blanket on top of the first one.

Variation: Ardha Supta Virasana

Supta Virasana & Ardha Supta Virasana
Reclined Hero's Pose • Half Reclined Hero's Pose

This restorative pose deeply opens the front of the body, ankles, quadriceps, hip flexors, and chest, and creates space in the abdomen, making it helpful for digestive complaints. It also eases morning sickness and lessens shortness of breath.

NOTE

For added comfort you can spread an additional blanket on the floor under your shins and feet. You should not feel pain in the knees or low back.

GETTING INTO THE POSE

1. Place a Narrow Fold blanket (p. 6) near the back of the sticky mat; place a block at the edge of the blanket and place one end of a bolster on the block; have about ½ foot between the edge of the blanket and the lower end of the bolster.
2. Kneel in front of the props, facing away from them; have the feet on either side of the narrow sides of the blanket and the big toes pointing straight back.
3. Take hold of the calves right behind the knees and roll the flesh of the calves out, away from the midline, and back toward the feet.
4. Sit down on the blanket, leaving a little space between the buttock and the bolster.
5. Roll the calves out to the sides away from the midline and draw the ankles in.
6. Spread your toes and press the little toes to the floor with your hands.
7. Lift and broaden the chest and then lower your back to the bolster.

ENGAGING ACTIONS

1. Draw the shoulders away from the ears to open the chest; tuck the shoulder blades into the back to open the chest further.
2. Release the groins and tops of the thighs down; there is a slight arch in the low back.

3. Close your eyes and soften the entire surface of the face.
4. Let the eyes retreat deep into the skull.
5. Let the lower jaw release completely from the upper jaw.
6. Observe your breath and find quietness.

Stay for a few minutes and for as long as you'd like.

COMING OUT OF THE POSE

1. Exhale; press the hands down by the sides.
2. Inhale; keeping the chest lifted, lead with the heart to come up to sitting.
3. Come to hands and knees, then push up into Adho Mukha Svanasana (p. 69) to open the back of the knees.

VARIATION: ARMS OVERHEAD

(not shown)

This variation brings extra length and openness to the side body.

1. In the pose, stretch your arms over your head and clasp your elbows.
2. Extend the arms strongly away from you to stretch the side body.
3. Stay for 5–10 breaths.

VARIATION: ARDHA SUPTA VIRASANA

Before lowering onto the bolster, extend one leg out and then proceed with the instructions for Supta Virasana.

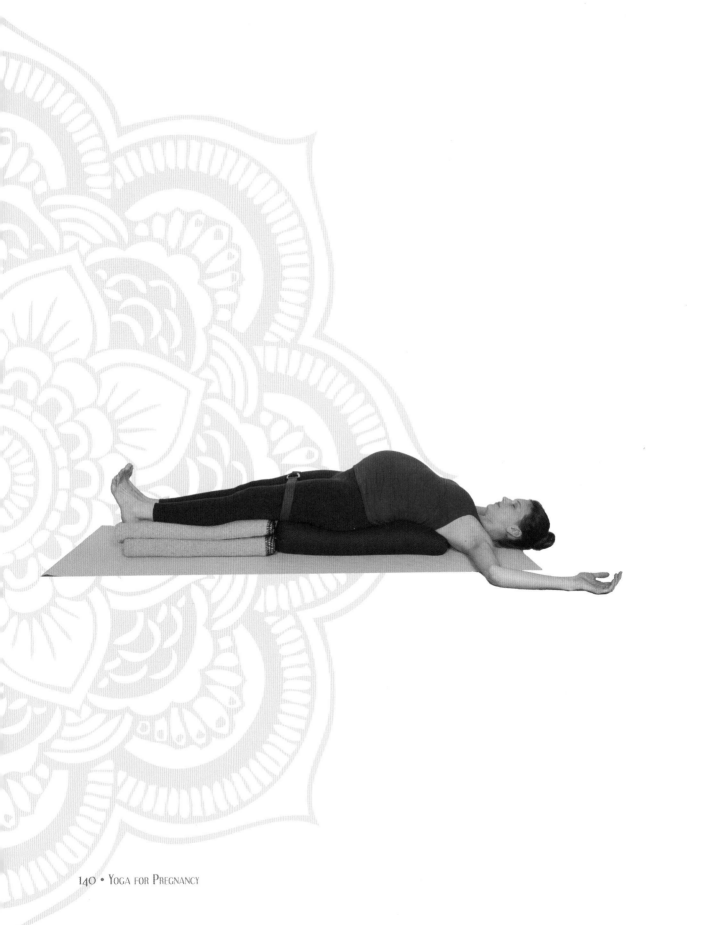

Setu Bandha Sarvangasana Restorative

Restorative Bridge Pose

Like many of the restoratives, this pose brings a sense of clarity and calmness. It opens the heart and refreshes the body in much the same way as the deep back bends that cannot be practiced during pregnancy. It reduces swelling in the legs and relieves fatigue.

Note

This is also a great pose to practice postpartum if you are breastfeeding, as it promotes healthy milk production.

Getting into the Pose

1. In the middle of your sticky mat, line up a bolster end to end with two blankets stacked on top of each other in Narrow Fold (p. 6).
2. Sit straddling the bolster, near the blankets.
3. Loop a belt around the mid-thighs; tighten the belt so that it is firm yet comfortable.
4. Keep the feet flat on the floor and lie back.
5. Scoot off of the bolster so the tops of the shoulders are on the sticky mat and the bottom tips of the shoulder blades are just at the edge of the bolster.
6. Point the fingers up to the ceiling and press the elbows down into the floor to open and broaden the chest, drawing the shoulder blades into the back body (see Pranayama Figure A, p. 155).
7. Bring your arms out to your sides and bend the elbows so they are in line with the shoulders and the hands are pointing away from your head. Move your sitting bones toward your heels to broaden and lengthen the low back.
8. Straighten your legs one by one onto the blankets.

Engaging Actions

1. Close your eyes and soften the entire surface of the face.
2. Let the eyes retreat deep into the skull.
3. Let the lower jaw release completely from the upper jaw.
4. Observe your breath and find quietness.

Note

If you are not comfortable in the pose, try adding 1–3 more blankets under the legs, so the legs are more elevated than your torso. In later stages of pregnancy, tighten the belt less and take the feet hip width apart or a bit wider.

Stay for at least a few minutes and for as long as you'd like.

Coming out of the Pose

1. Staying reclined, loosen the belt, and bring your feet to the floor on either side of the blankets.
2. Roll over to your side and pause here for several breaths before coming up to sitting.

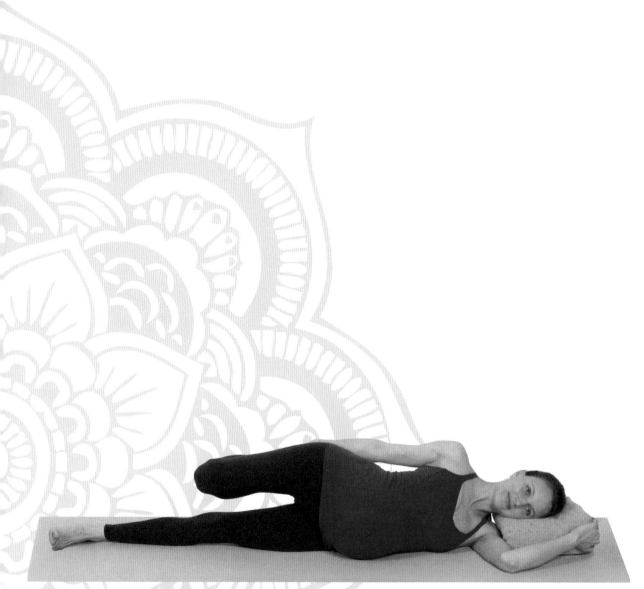

Side Lying Quadricep Stretch

This is a simple way to open the front of the thighs while resting.

Getting into the Pose

1. Place a blanket at the end of your mat in Side Lying Pillow Fold (p. 7).
2. Lie on the sticky mat on your left side, with your left ear on the blanket.
3. Bend your right knee and take hold of your ankle with your right hand.

Engaging Actions

1. Draw the tailbone in and the sitting bones down toward the backs of the knees.
2. Roll the right upper arm out and take the shoulder blades into the back to open and broaden the chest.
3. Exhale; press your right ankle into your right hand.
4. Inhale; move the sternum bone away from your navel.
5. Soften your eyes, relax your face, and let the breath flow freely.

Details to be Mindful of

Keep the thighs parallel to each other.

Stay for 5–10 breaths.

Coming out of the Pose

Release the bent leg and rest.

Repeat on the other side.

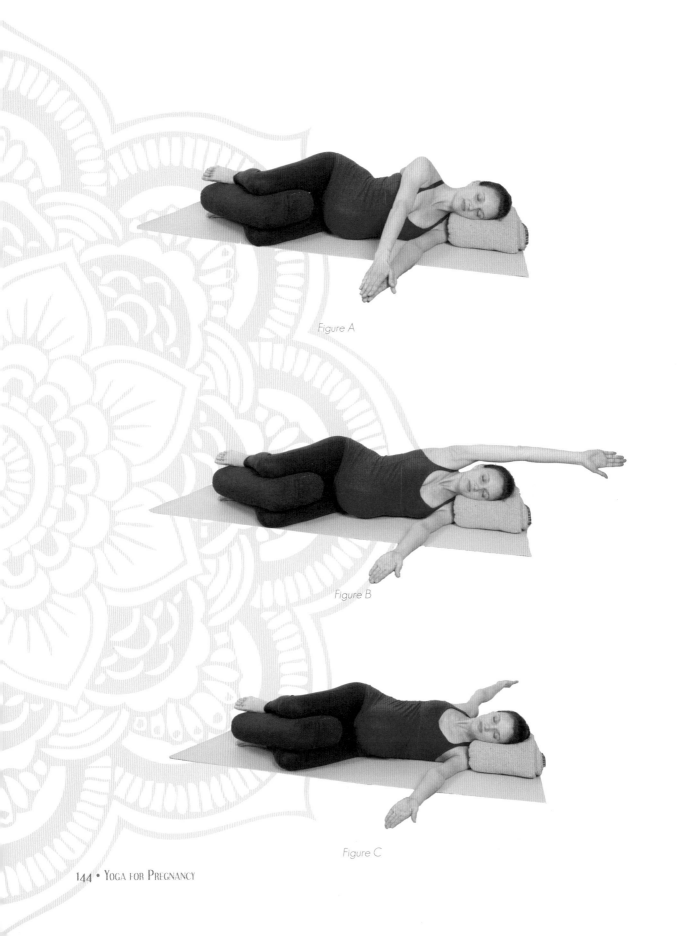

Figure A

Figure B

Figure C

Side Lying Arm Circles

This dynamic, restful pose works tension out of the upper back and shoulders.

GETTING INTO THE POSE

1. Start in side lying Savasana with bolster (Variation on p. 149).
2. Take both arms out in front of you on the floor in line with your chest; have the palms together (*Figure A*).
3. Keeping the chest open, reach through the fingertips to extend the arms fully and draw your shoulders back and down, away from your ears.
4. Exhale; relax your face, tongue, eyes, and throat.
5. Inhale; circle the right arm up over the head (*Figure B*).
6. Exhale; continue the circle by bringing the arm behind you (*Figure C*), down toward your hip, and then back around to the front, joining your other hand.

DETAILS TO BE MINDFUL OF

Let the movement be fluid.

Continue for 5–15 breaths, pausing for a few breaths to release tension in any areas that feel particularly tight.

Repeat on the other side.

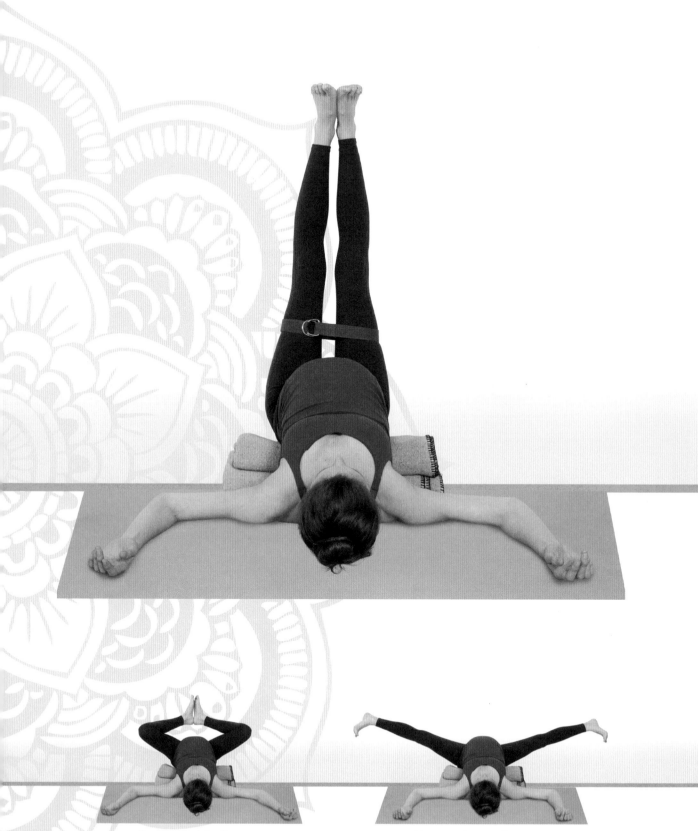

Variation: Baddha Konasana

Variation: Upavista Konasana

Viparita Karani
Inverted Seal Pose / Legs up the Wall Pose

This pose is helpful for decompressing from a stressful day. It relaxes the mind and body, relieves morning sickness, reduces swelling in the legs, can prevent varicose veins, and supports deep, restful sleep. It is a great pose to practice just before going to bed.

Getting into the pose

1. Place two blankets in Basic Fold 4–6 inches away from the wall.
2. Sit on the blankets with your right hip against the wall.
3. Place a loosely looped belt around your upper mid-thighs and tighten it up so it is snug yet comfortable.
4. Lie down on your left side and scoot your buttock to the wall.
5. Simultaneously swing your legs up against the wall and rotate your body so that both heels are on the wall and your back is on the floor. Have the buttock just off the blankets toward the wall so there is a slight arch in the low back.
6. Bring your arms out to your sides and bend the elbows so they are in line with the shoulders and the hands are slightly above your head.

Engaging actions

1. Draw the shoulders away from the ears to open the chest; tuck the shoulder blades into the back to open the chest further.
2. Relax the inner groin down.
3. Close your eyes and soften the entire surface of the face.
4. Let the eyes retreat deep into the skull.
5. Let the lower jaw release completely from the upper jaw.
6. Observe your breath and find quietness.

Note

If you experience any discomfort in your low back, try removing a blanket. Conversely, if you have a long torso, you may want to add an extra blanket in order to get more opening in the chest. If you have sacral issues, you may be most comfortable with the buttock on less height.

In later stages of pregnancy, widen the feet to hip width to accommodate the belly.

Stay for at least a few minutes and for as long as you'd like.

Variation: Baddha Konasana

Prior to coming out of the pose, remove the belt and bring the feet together into Baddha Konasana (p. 93). You can either come out of the pose or proceed to Upavista Konasana Variation (p. 95).

Variation: Upavista Konasana

Prior to coming out of the pose, remove the belt and take the legs wide into Upavista Konasana (p. 95).

Coming out of the pose

Bend the knees, loosen the belt (if you haven't already removed it), and roll to the side; pause here for a few breaths and then come up to sitting.

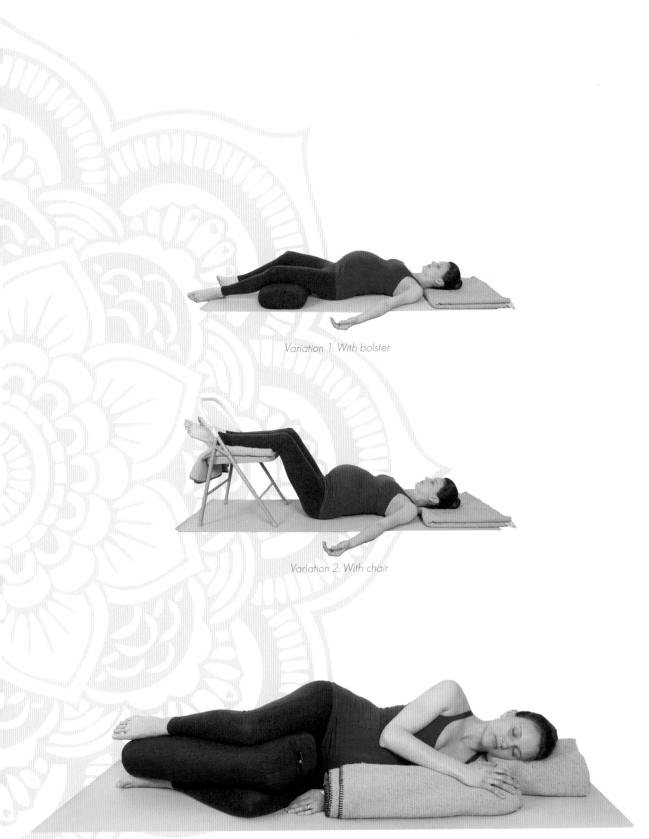

Variation 1: With bolster

Variation 2: With chair

Variation 3: Side lying with bolster

Savasana
Corpse Pose

This is a very important pose and some variation of it should always be included at the end of your practice. It is essential for allowing you to fully absorb the benefits of your practice and finish feeling peaceful.

NOTE

The variations presented here are designed to support the body during pregnancy, when lying flat on your back (as in the classic pose) is not comfortable.

VARIATION 1: WITH BOLSTER

1. Place a blanket in Open Fold (p. 6) at one end of your sticky mat.
2. Lay a bolster 1–2 feet from the other end of the mat.
3. Lie down so that the head and neck (but not the shoulders) are on the blanket and the bolster is under the knees.
4. Draw your shoulders away from your ears.
5. Move your sitting bones toward your heels to broaden and lengthen the low back.
6. Close your eyes and soften the entire surface of the face.
7. Let the eyes retreat deep into the skull.
8. Let the lower jaw release completely from the upper jaw.
9. Observe your breath and find quietness.
10. Stay for at least 5 minutes and as long as you want.

COMING OUT OF THE POSE

Roll to your right side and pause for a few breaths; then, staying quiet inside, come up to sitting.

VARIATION 2: WITH CHAIR

1. Place a blanket in Open Fold at one end of your sticky mat.
2. Place a chair at the other end of your mat, with a blanket lying over the seat in Open Fold.
3. Lie down so that the head and neck (but not the shoulders) are on the blanket and your calves are resting on the seat on the chair.
4. Follow steps 4–10 from Variation #1.

VARIATION 3: SIDE LYING WITH BOLSTER

1. Place a blanket in Pillow Fold (p. 7) at one end of your sticky mat.
2. Have a bolster and a rolled blanket (p. 6) within reach.
3. Lie down on your side and bend your knees slightly.
4. Bring the bolster between the legs so that it is supporting your knees, ankles, and feet.
5. Rest your top arm on the rolled blanket to keep your chest open.
6. Follow steps 4–10 from Variation #1.

continued on next page

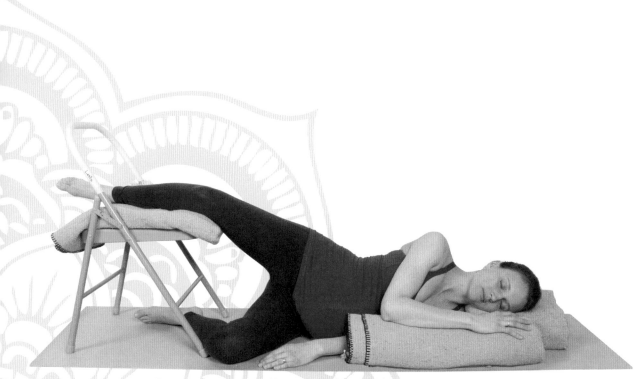

Variation 4: Side lying with chair

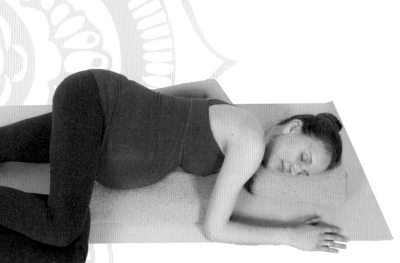

Variation 5: Side lying with bolster and rotated arms

VARIATION 4: SIDE LYING WITH CHAIR

1. Place a blanket in Pillow Fold (p. 7) at one end of your sticky mat.
2. Place a chair at the other end of your mat, with a blanket lying over the seat in Basic Fold.
3. Have a rolled blanket within reach.
4. Lie down on your side and bend your knees slightly; rest your top shin on the chair.
5. Rest your top arm on the rolled blanket to keep your chest open.
6. Follow steps 4–10 from Variation #1.

VARIATION 5: SIDE LYING WITH BOLSTER AND ROTATED ARMS

1. Place a blanket in Basic Fold (p. 6) at one end of your sticky mat.
2. Have a Narrow Fold blanket (p. 6) nearby.
3. Place a bolster at the other end of the mat.
4. Lie down on your side and bend the top leg to rest it on the bolster; adjust as needed so that the knee, lower leg, and ankle are all supported.
5. Rotate the bottom shoulder so the fingers are pointing down toward your feet; bend your top arm so that the fingers point toward your head.
6. If it feels comfortable, slide the Narrow Fold blanket underneath the belly to support baby.
7. Follow steps 4–10 from Variation #1.

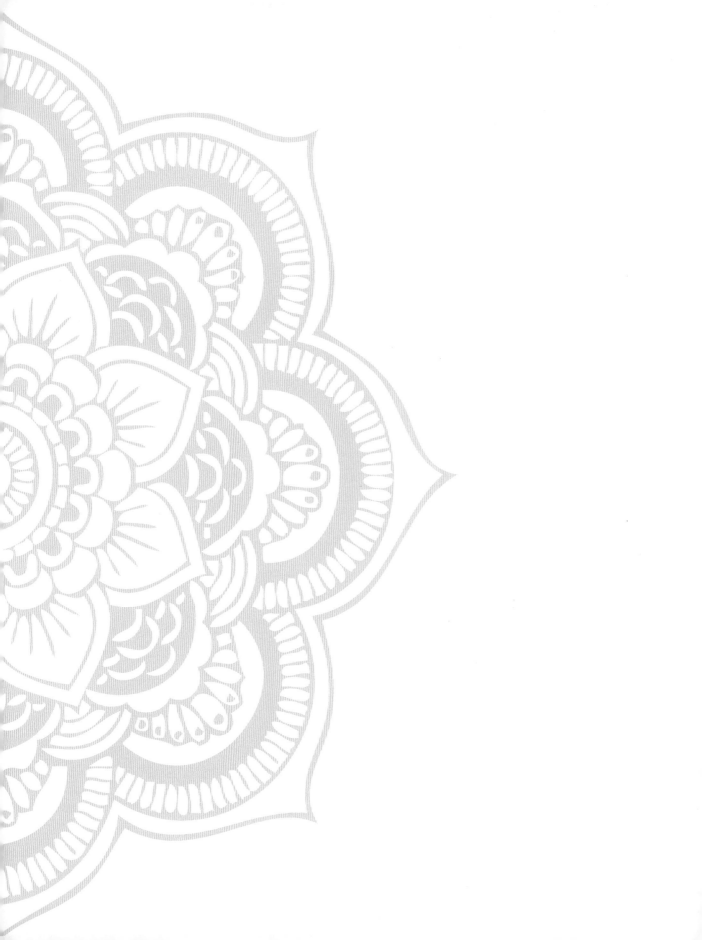

PRANAYAMA

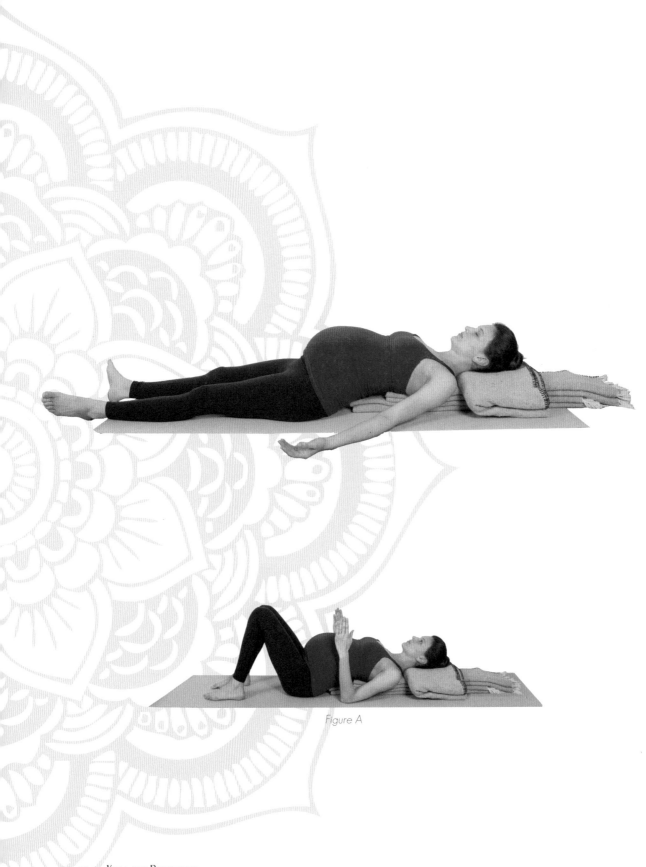

Figure A

Pranayama

"Prana" means "life force" in Sanskrit; "pranayama" is the refined control of life force through mindful breathing. Pranayama practice develops the ability to breathe fully and deeply, which has profound physical and mental benefits. These yogic breathing techniques massage the organs and calm the nervous system.

Practice pranayama after Savasana. After pranayama, practice Savasana again.

Note

During the practice of pranayama you want the breath to be smooth and soft at all times. If the breath becomes labored, feels forced, or you feel anxiety or strain, discontinue the technique and return to your normal breathing. If after some time with normal breathing you feel able to return to the technique, then do so. If the breath again becomes strained or labored, discontinue for the day and practice Savasana. It is extremely helpful to have a qualified teacher guide you in practicing pranayama. Be sure that you do not strain the breath in any way.

Preparing for Pranayama

1. Have two blankets in Narrow Trifold (p. 7); place the first blanket toward the back of the sticky mat and have the second blanket on top of the first, staggered back about 3–4 inches.

2. Place a blanket in Basic Fold horizontally across the other blankets; this blanket will be used as a pillow.

3. Sit a few inches in front of the bottom blanket and lie back; see that the edge of the bottom blanket is under the mid to low back and the top blanket is right under the chest, so it facilitates your chest being open and ready to receive the breath.

4. Move the Basic Fold blanket so the base of the blanket goes right to the base of the neck; the shoulders are not on this blanket.

5. See that the forehead is slightly higher than the chest and the belly is lower than the chest.

6. Point your fingers up to the ceiling and press your elbows down to the floor and lift your chest up higher. Draw the tips of the shoulder blades into the back to open the chest more (*Figure A*).

7. Keeping the chest open, relax your arms by your sides, palms facing up.

8. Straighten your legs; draw your sit bones to the back of the knees to broaden and lengthen your low back.

9. Soften your face completely.

10. Close your eyes and draw the eyes back into the sockets.

11. Let the eyes be still; you can place an eye pillow over the eyes to encourage stillness.

12. Relax your tongue and the lower jaw.

13. Allow your mind to be passive yet alert.

continued on next page

Pranayama

Pranayama Technique 1: Ujjayi I

Ujjayi can be translated as "upward, expanding, conquest, success, victory." It is the very beginning stage of pranayama. In this stage we observe the steady passing of the exhale and the inhale and focus on smoothing out any tension.

1. Exhale completely (this is always the first step when beginning pranayama practice). Let your breath be gentle without any force—smooth and steady.

2. To inhale, take a smooth, steady, slow inhalation in through the inner walls of the nostrils. As you are inhaling, observe the chest filling slowly and equally in the front, sides, and backs of the ribs. Expand the ribs from the sternum outward to the sides as well as upward. Expand the breath equally throughout the inhale. During the inhalation, observe the sound "ssss."

3. After a full, slow inhalation there may be a natural pause that occurs. If so, allow this pause to happen effortlessly for a few seconds.

4. Then, when the body is naturally ready, exhale a nice slow, soft, steady exhalation out through the outer walls of the nostrils. Keep the mind and eyes still. Keep the throat and entire face relaxed. As you exhale, let the lift and expansion of the chest release slowly, smoothly, and gradually, just like the breath. Observe the sound "hhhh" as you exhale.

5. Again, you may observe a natural pause after the end of the exhalation.

6. After that pause, begin again with the inhalation and continue the cycle.

7. Continue this practice for a few minutes at first and then build the practice to 5–15 minutes daily.

Details to be mindful of:

As you breathe in and out, fill and empty the lungs evenly. If you notice unevenness, use your awareness correct it.

Pranayama

PRANAYAMA TECHNIQUE 2: UJJAYI II

In this stage of Ujjayi, we take a normal steady inhalation and lengthen the exhalation. This stage helps to relax physical, mental, and emotional tension. It is a quieting pranayama.

1. Begin with a smooth, steady, even exhalation to empty the lungs completely and slowly, without force.
2. Inhale normally through the nose, paying close attention to the subtleties of your breath, lungs, and the flow of air into the nostrils.
3. Allow a natural pause in between the inhalation and exhalation.
4. Now exhale slowly, breathing out through the nose. Let the breath be long and slow. Feel the lungs emptying equally. When the lungs are empty, again allow for a natural pause before taking a normal inhalation.
5. Continue this practice for a few minutes at first and then build the practice to 5–15 minutes daily.

NOTE

To help keep the breathing relaxed and unlabored, try taking 1–3 normal breath cycles (inhalation and exhalations) in between the long exhalation and the normal inhalation.

PRANAYAMA TECHNIQUE 3: VILOMA I

Viloma can be translated as "against the hair" or "against the natural order of things."

In Viloma pranayama the inhalation and exhalations are broken into parts rather than being one continuous stream of breath.

In the first stage of Viloma, we break the inhalation into parts and have one even, continuous exhalation. This is an energizing pranayama.

1. Begin by practicing Ujjayi I for a few minutes or longer.
2. Next, do a few rounds of normal breathing.
3. Exhale.
4. As you take a smooth, steady inhalation, imagine your chest and ribs are like a pear-shaped vessel. First fill and expand the bottom third of the vessel, using about a third of the capacity of your inhalation. Expand the lower ribs out to the sides and outward toward the ceiling. Coordinate evenness throughout the chest. Pause for a few seconds. Then, fill the middle of the vessel, again simultaneously expanding the ribs and chest area up toward the ceiling and out to the sides. Pause for a few seconds. Now, using the last third of the inhalation, breathe into the top of the vessel, again expanding up and out to the sides simultaneously.
5. Pause.
6. Now, slowly, softly, and evenly exhale completely.
7. Take 1–3 normal breaths and then repeat steps 4–6.
8. Practice this pranayama for 5 or so minutes and then rest in Savasana for at least 5 minutes.

PRACTICING KEGELS

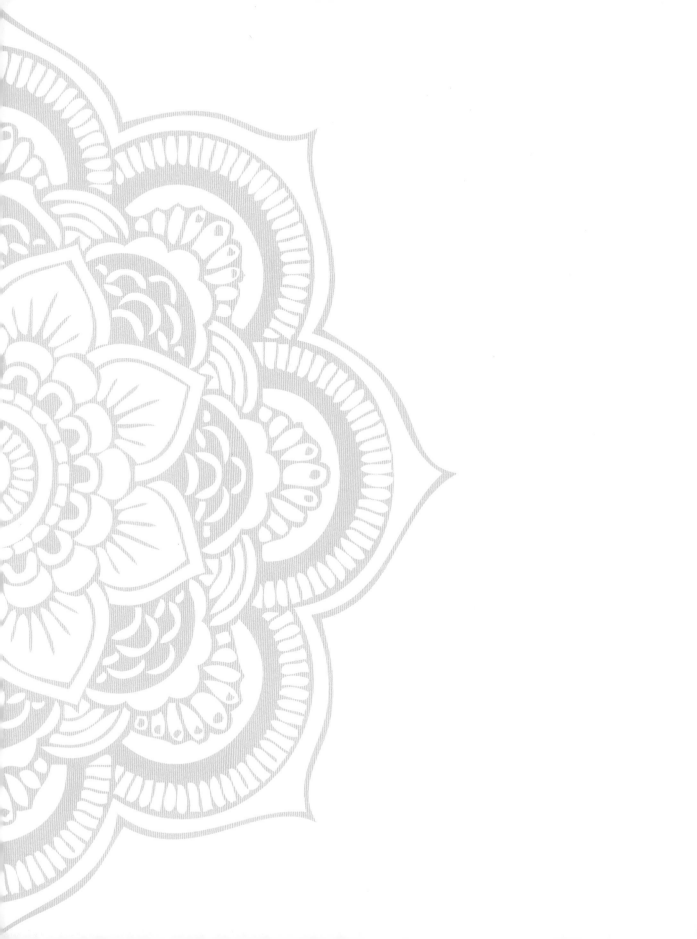

Practicing Kegels

Doing Kegels during your pregnancy and especially postpartum is a fantastic practice. Kegels strengthen the "hammock" of the pelvic floor muscles, remedying urinary incontinence and encouraging the abdominal organs to remain in a healthy place. Pregnancy and birth can cause the pelvic floor to become stretched and lax, which can lead pelvic organs, like the uterus, to sag or prolapse. The daily practice of Kegels throughout pregnancy and postpartum is extremely valuable.

You can practice Kegels anywhere: in your car, at work, while breastfeeding your baby, or during your yoga practice. No one can tell you are doing them. It is ideal to do 200 a day, which is a lot. At first, see if you can do 20 a day, then maybe 50, and then work your way up to 200. Quality is better than quantity. Really focus on each Kegel and take time to create the correct actions. Do what you can; a few Kegels is better than no Kegels.

To do Kegels

1. Start with an empty bladder.
2. Exhale fully; inhale and draw the pelvic floor up by contracting the muscles that you would use to stop the flow of urine midstream. If you are unsure of how to do this, practice while urinating and see if you have the correct action. It is a lifting and squeezing-up action.
3. Hold this pelvic floor lift for the full inhalation and then release with your exhalation. If doing the exercise properly you will not feel the buttock, legs, or abdominal muscles contract.
4. Keep your breath flowing while you practice.

Note

You can also try holding the pelvic floor lift for multiple breaths, retaining the contraction while you inhale and exhale. Then, take a few resting breaths and again hold the Kegel for multiple breaths.

This practice of holding the action for multiple breaths can be done every 5 breaths. For example, for Kegel 1, 2, 3, and 4 you are contracting as you inhale and releasing with your exhale. Then for the 5th Kegel, you can hold the action for multiple breaths as described above. Continue Kegel number 6, 7, 8, and 9 with the hold just for a single inhalation, and so on.

Some poses that are great to add Kegels to are Supta Baddha Konasana (p. 135); Upavista Konasana (p. 95), Half Squat (p. 57); Squat Variations (p. 59); and Baddha Konasana (p. 93).

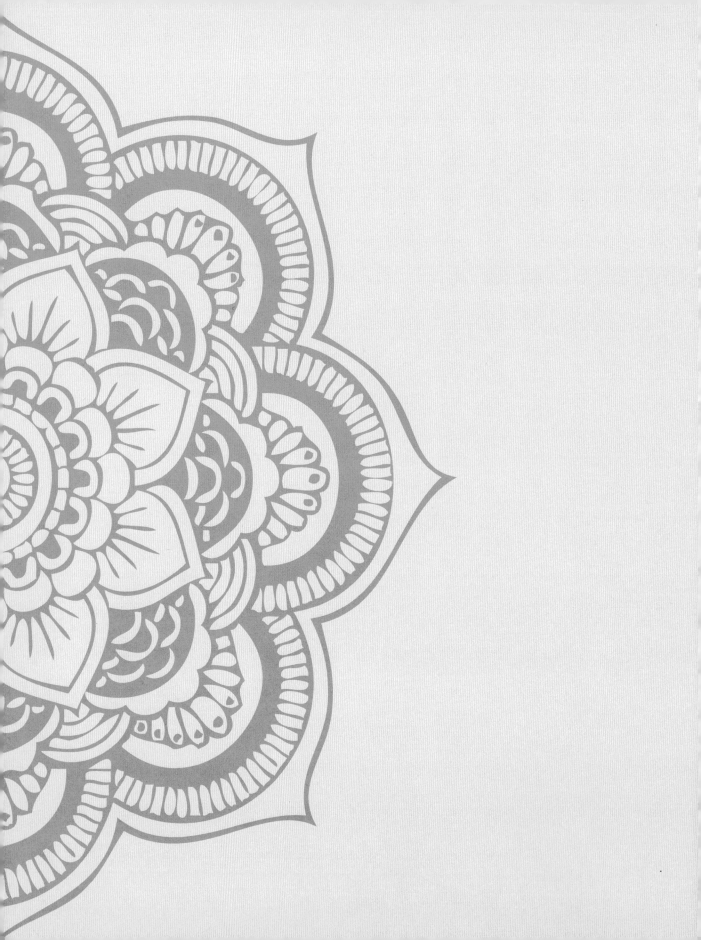

Inspiration and Sequences

The anatomy of yoga includes subtle energy bodies in addition to the physical body.

Chakras are psycho-energetic vortexes in the subtle body. There are seven of them, aligned vertically along the core of the physical axial body from the perineum to the crown of the head. These wheels of energy correspond to the physiological nerve plexuses.

Bringing consciousness to the chakras is a powerful way to refine and strengthen your life force *(prana)* in order to experience greater ease and skillfulness as a human being—and as a mother. This section of the book is organized around the seven chakras. For each chakra, we include a suite of tools to help you access and engage your subtle energy body.

ॐ MANTRA

Chanting mantras is a form of *bhakti*, or devotional, yoga. Mantra practice can be a lovely way to cleanse and refresh your heart and spirit. This is especially valuable during times in your pregnancy when you feel tired and in need of a quick reset.

👁 VISUALIZATION

The guidance in this section is designed to help you cultivate an ability to see the chakras in your mind's eye. This in turn can help you to connect more tangibly with your subtle energy body.

🫖 TEA RECIPES

How you nourish yourself with food and drink is so important during pregnancy. While we will leave the details to another book, please remember how important it is to avoid pesticides, chemicals and genetically modified organisms during pregnancy. Look for certified organic and Non-GMO Project Verified choices when you shop.

In this section, we couldn't resist sharing some tidbits from Leslie's work as an herbalist. Blending your own teas is a fun project and can also make a wonderful gift for pregnant friends. Note that the recipes are given in "parts"; a part can be measured in ounces, spoonfuls, or whatever works for you. If you have left over herb mixtures, store herbs in a cool, dark and dry place to retain the potency of the herbs.

📖 REFLECTION AND PRACTICE

Quiet contemplation and self-reflection are important elements of a yoga practice. The reflection prompts offered here delve into different aspects of experience related to each chakra and to the journey of pregnancy.

🧘 MEDITATION

The meditations in this section are practices from the *Kundalini Yoga* tradition. Most of them involve subtle, repetitive movements to develop awareness, consciousness, and spiritual strength. If you are inspired to learn more about these practices, check out Gurmukh Kaur Khalsa's book *Bountiful, Beautiful, Blissful* (details in Resources and References, p. 279).

⚙ SEQUENCES

Finally, we have developed posture sequences that use the physical body to access the subtle body and activate each chakra.

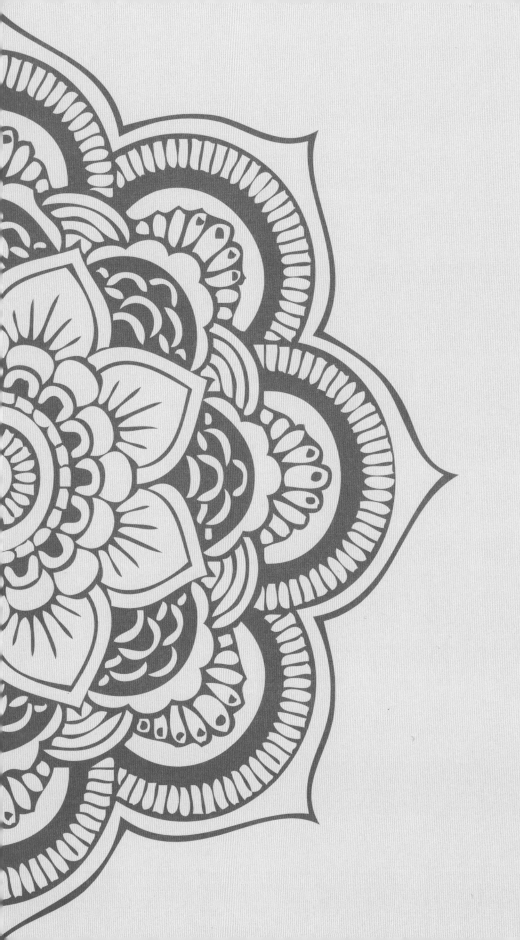

● Grounded
ROOT CHAKRA (Muladhara) मूलाधार

The root chakra, *muladhara*, is our energetic foundation, and when it is balanced it brings a grounded quality full of strength, stability, and security. Ruled by the earth element, the root chakra is concerned with basic survival and material needs like food and shelter.

During pregnancy, this relates strongly to the "nesting instinct" that commonly kicks in toward the end of the third trimester. As you prepare your physical space for the arrival of baby, you nourish your *muladhara* chakra and bring a fundamental sense of groundedness into the most basic level of your being.

The root chakra is also a powerful energy center during labor. Many of the poses that help labor progress are full of root gravity, bringing the weight of the body deeply toward the firm support of the earth.

ॐ Mantra

As the first chakra, *muladhara* is also associated with a quality of innocence, and is ruled by Ganesha, the elephant-headed deity who is the god of beginnings, the eternal child, and the remover of obstacles. Also known as Ganapati, Ganesh represents the pure, childlike joy that resides within each of us. This quality is often compromised by material realm insecurity, such as financial stress or other fears related to basic survival. Chanting this invocation helps clear such obstacles from our perception, allowing us to experience the innocent delight that is our birthright.

Connecting with the qualities of Ganesha is wonderful preparation for aligning with the unencumbered purity that your sweet baby will be born embodying.

Om Gam Ganapataye Namaha

Pronunciation

Om = ohm

Gam = gahm

Ganapateye = gan-ah-pah-tah-YAY

Namaha = nam-ah-ha

For inspiration, check out MC Yogi's album Elephant Power; the track "Elephant Power (feat. Bhagavan Das)" features this mantra.

�👁 Visualization

Settle into a comfortable, reclined position, such as Savasana (p. 149). Close your eyes and bring your awareness to the bottom of your torso. Envision a glowing sphere of deep red energy surrounding the base of your spine, your perineum, and your pubic bone. Imagine this energy spreading through your legs like roots of a tree, stabilizing you and connecting you with the earth. Feel how the ground is supporting you and your baby unconditionally; let yourself be heavy, melting into gravity completely.

● Grounded
ROOT CHAKRA (Muladhara) मूलाधार

🫖 Mama and Baby Nutritive Tea

This tea is packed with vitamins and minerals to nourish you and the baby inside you.

2 parts nettles

2 parts raspberry leaf

2 parts oatstraw

1 part mint

1 part dandelion root

Place 2 teaspoons of the above mixture in a cup or jar. Pour 1 cup hot water over it and steep for at least 20 minutes and as long as overnight. Longer steeping extracts more minerals from the herbs and is more nutritious.

Strain and enjoy. Drink up to 3 cups a day hot or cold.

📖 Reflection & Practice

What makes you feel grounded? When do you feel the most firmly settled and solid in your body and being? Is there a particular place, person, or activity that helps give you a sense of stability? Once you've thought of something, take a moment to close your eyes and really experience the sense of safety you get from that person or thing. Create a sense memory that you can keep returning to during your pregnancy and labor—a touch point of security to help you come back to a place of groundedness and support. With practice, this feeling is something you can access and create for yourself no matter what is going on around you.

⚜ MEDITATION FOR REMOVING OBSTACLES

1. Sit in a comfortable cross-legged position, with enough blankets under you so that your knees drop down to the height of your hips or lower.

2. Close your eyes and roll them upward.

3. Sit up tall and lift from the crown of your head, lengthening your spine and tucking your chin slightly.

4. Stretch your arms straight out to either side so that they are parallel with the ground.

5. Close your hands so that the tips of your fingers touch the base of your palms and your thumbs point upward.

6. As you inhale, bend at the elbows to bring your thumbs as close to your shoulders as possible without actually touching them (*Figure A*).

7. Exhale as you extend your arms and bring your hands back to their starting position.

8. Repeat for two minutes with strong, even breaths.

Figure A

◉ Grounded Sequence
ROOT CHAKRA (Muladhara) मूलाधार

During the following sequence, pay special attention to your connection with the ground. Feel the solidity of the earth supporting your feet, hands, and legs as you move through the poses. Let that grounded energy radiate up through your body and infuse you with stability.

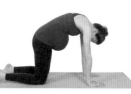

1. Cat (p. 119)

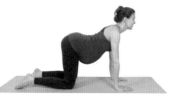

2. Cow (p. 119)

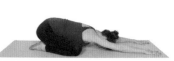

3. Adho Mukha Virasana (p. 107)

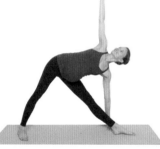

7. Utthita Trikonasana (p. 33)
(Both sides)

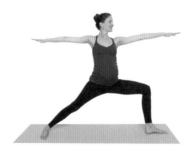

8. Virabhadrasana II (p. 35)
(Both sides)

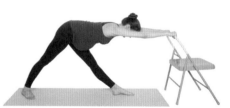

9. Parsvottanasana (hands to chair) (p. 44)
(Both sides)

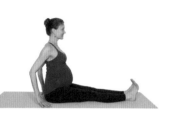

13. Dandasana (p. 77)

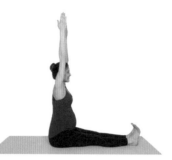

14. Urdhva Hasta Dandasana (p. 79)

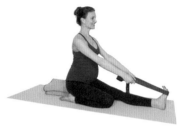

15. Triang Mukhaikapada
Paschimottanasana (p. 89)
(Both sides)

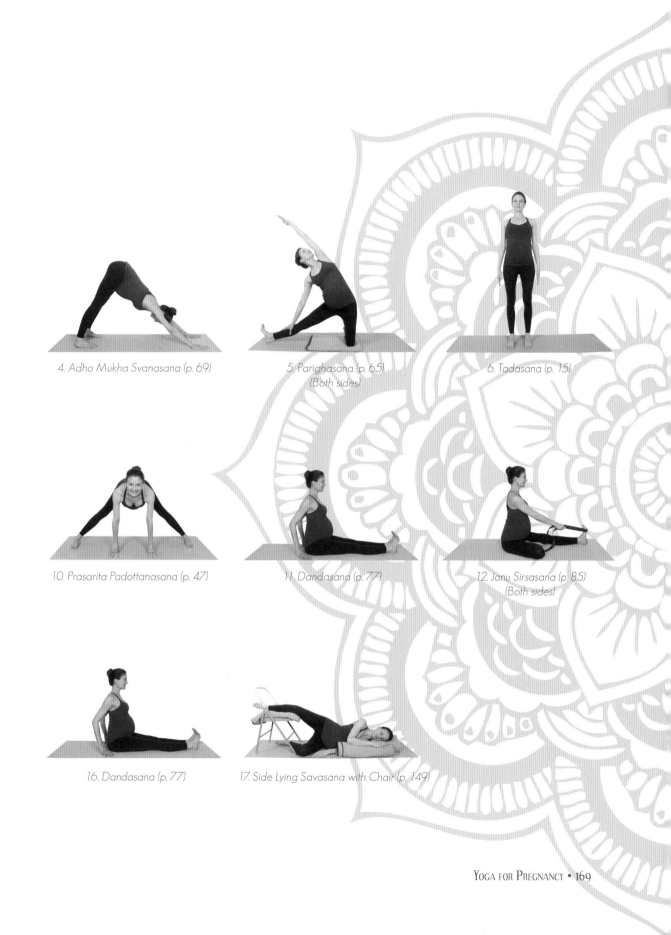

4. Adho Mukha Svanasana (p. 69)

5. Parighasana (p. 65)
(Both sides)

6. Tadasana (p. 15)

10. Prasarita Padottanasana (p. 47)

11. Dandasana (p. 77)

12. Janu Sirsasana (p. 85)
(Both sides)

16. Dandasana (p. 77)

17. Side Lying Savasana with Chair (p. 149)

Creative
BELLY CHAKRA (Svadhisthana) स्वाधिष्ठान

As the source of all creativity, the belly chakra, *svadhisthana*, is especially powerful during pregnancy. From the belly chakra comes our ability to feel a healthy connection to our own sensuality, fertility, and capacity for creative production of all kinds . . . including the miraculous ability to grow a human being!

The belly chakra is ruled by the water element, from which all life comes. At birth, humans are 75–78 percent water, and by adulthood most people's bodies are around 60 percent water. Pure, clean water is essential to our basic functioning. We typically don't feel dehydrated until our bodies have lost 2–3 percent of their water, but at only 1 percent water loss we have already begun to suffer from reduced physical and mental function.

Drinking lots of filtered water is always important, but this is especially true during pregnancy when it is recommended to drink at least eight 8-ounce glasses a day (64 ounces total), plus an additional 8 ounces for every hour of exercise. Drinking plenty of fluids can help ease two common discomforts of pregnancy, constipation and leg cramps, and can also help prevent premature labor. Drinking water is also essential during labor. Staying well-hydrated leading up to and during your baby's birth can really help the process flow (literally!). Finally, especially if you're breastfeeding, drinking lots of water is also extremely helpful postpartum. It takes a lot of water to make all that milk!

The belly chakra is also associated with emotions, which can flow through us with special intensity during the journey of pregnancy. Balancing the belly chakra can help harness emotional energy and teach us to be more at peace with the ups and downs of this transformative time.

ॐ MANTRA

Vishnu, the lord of preservation, is the deity associated with the belly chakra. Vishnu, who also appears as the avatars Ram and Krishna, is often shown with blue skin. This blue symbolizes that, like the sky or ocean, Vishnu has a borderless, vast quality.

Chanting to Vishnu reminds us of the vastness within ourselves. From the infinite and unknowable expanse inside us comes our miraculous ability to create and sustain life.

Om Namo Bhagavate Vasudevaya

Pronunciation

Om = ohm

Namo = nahm-oh

Bhagavate = bah-gah-vah-tay

Vasudevaya = vas-oo-day-vie-yah

For inspiration, check out Deva Premal's album Deva Premal's Healing Mantras; the track "Om Namo Bhagavate Vasudevaya" features this mantra.

👁 VISUALIZATION

Settle into a comfortable, reclined position, such as *Supta Badha Konasana* (p. 131). Close your eyes and bring your awareness to your belly. If you like, rest your hands gently on either side of your belly button, just over where your baby is growing. Envision a glowing sphere of vibrant orange energy surrounding your lower abdomen and low back. Imagine this energy holding your precious baby in its light. Feel your own vast capacity for creativity and sustenance; let yourself silently hum with the glow of fertility and sensuality.

⊙ Creative
BELLY CHAKRA (Svadhisthana) स्वाधिष्ठान

🫖 Postpartum Sitz Bath Tea

This is a bath tea, for external application after birth. **It is not a tea for drinking.**

2 parts sage

2 parts lavender

1 part witch hazel

2 parts white oak bark

1 part rose petals

3 parts calendula flowers

3 parts comfrey leaves

Mix all the herbs in a large bowl. It would be ideal to end up with 1–2 cups of the final sitz bath blend. After baby is born, have someone brew this blend for you by placing 8 tablespoons of the herb mixture in 4 cups of hot water and stirring. Place a lid on the pot. Let steep for at least 30 minutes and as long as 8 hours. (This is a great activity for someone to do for you while you are in labor.) Strain and refrigerate for up to 3 days.

When you are ready to use the tea, be sure that the tea has cooled to room temperature. Place the tea in a peri bottle and leave near the toilet. Squeeze the bottle so the tea washes over your perineum and vaginal tissues each time you use the restroom, to promote healing. This also **real**ly helps ease the stinging that occurs postpartum when there is tearing from birth.

You can also prepare this tea ahead of time and place a postpartum pad in a bowl. Pour the tea over the pad and place in a freezer. Do this for a few pads. To remove from the bowl postpartum, turn the bowl over and run hot water over the bottom of the bowl. After birth you can use them as an ice pack (be sure to have a towel over the pad so when it melts it doesn't get your bed wet).

The sitz bath tea can also be added to bath water.

📖 Reflection & Practice

Pregnancy and the first weeks and months postpartum can be a roller coaster of emotions. Much of this is due to rapid and dramatic hormonal fluctuations, but with intention and practice it is possible to keep from feeling overrun by emotions. The following practice is adapted from an exercise called "Riding the Wave,"[1] which was developed by Stephen Cope, a yoga scholar at the Kripalu Center in Massachusetts.

The concept here is that we are not our emotions, no matter how powerful and consuming they can feel. Through practice we can learn to fully experience our emotions without becoming mired in them.

Breathe. As you notice an emotion arising, connect to your breath. Breathe slowly and deeply.

Relax. Soften your belly, your face, and your shoulders. Actively find softness in your body.

Feel. Notice any place in your body that is tensing up in response to the emotion, and release it with an exhale. Observe how the emotion you are experiencing feels in your body, and move toward the sensations rather than away from them.

Watch. As you breathe, relax, and feel, connect with the part of yourself that can observe the experience, the witness consciousness quietly watching from the core of your being. This witness is always present and always available to you.

Allow. Stay with your experience, and know that it is safe to make space for whatever you are feeling. If you feel yourself starting to resist, return to the breath, to relaxation, and use those as tools for allowing the emotion to move through you as you witness from a place of compassion.

---

1   Riding the Wave exercise is from Stephen Cope's CD "Yoga for Emotional Flow." The same practice is described in depth in Cope's book The Wisdom of Yoga.

♨ Meditation for Emotional Balance

1. Sit in a comfortable cross-legged position, with enough blankets under you so that your knees drop down to the height of your hips or lower.

2. Close your eyes and roll them upward.

3. Sit up tall and lift from the crown of your head, lengthening your spine.

4. Reach your arms straight up toward the sky, with palms turned toward each other. Keep the fingers of each hand pressed together, with the thumbs separate.

5. Repetitively fan your arms in and out, moving about six inches out and back in each time (*Figure A*).

6. Repeat for three minutes with relaxed, even breaths.

Figure A

◉ Creative Sequence
BELLY CHAKRA (Svadhisthana) स्वाधिष्ठान

When you are in Adho Mukha Virasana, enjoy the experience of bowing with humble surrender. You can use this pose as preparation for labor; imagine it as the break between contractions in which you can rest and find your strength. Practice utilizing your breath to quickly and deeply find quietness and peace before returning to activity.

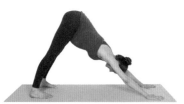

1. Baddha Konasana (p. 93)

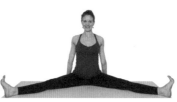

2. Upavista Konasana (p. 95)

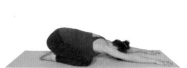

3. Seated Window Stretch (p. 99)
(Both sides)

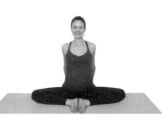

7. Adho Mukha Svanasana (p. 69)

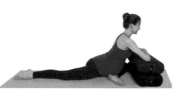

8. Eka Pada Rajakapotanasana (p. 123)
(Both sides)

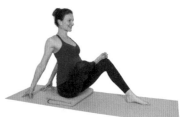

9. Adho Mukha Virasana (p. 107)

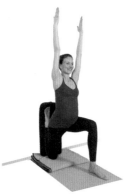

13. Half Lunge at Wall (p. 63)
(Both sides)

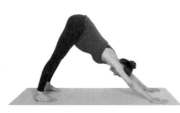

14. Adho Mukha Svanasana (p. 69)

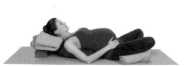

15. Supta Svastikasana (p. 137)

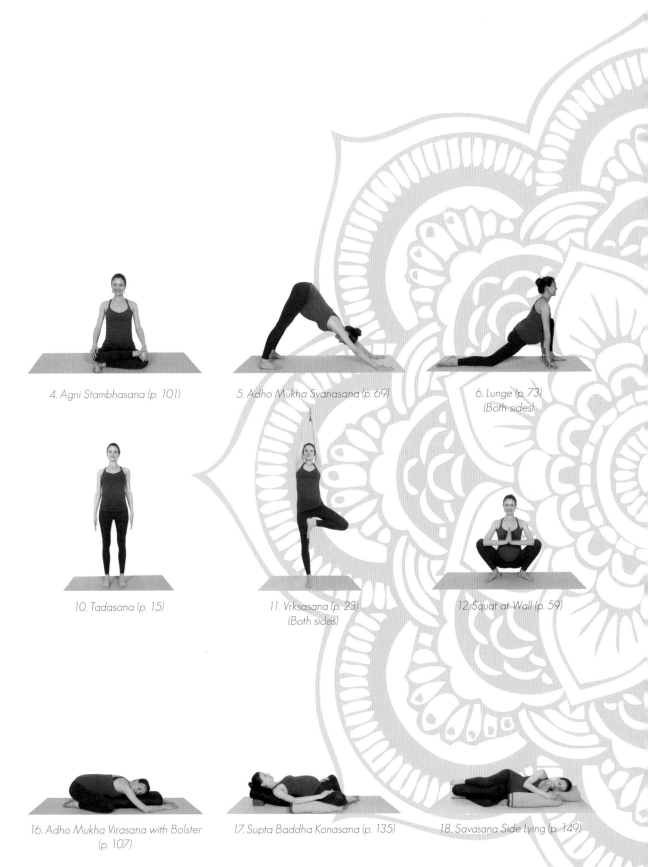

4. Agni Stambhasana (p. 101)

5. Adho Mukha Svanasana (p. 69)

6. Lunge (p. 73)
(Both sides)

10. Tadasana (p. 15)

11. Vrksasana (p. 23)
(Both sides)

12. Squat at Wall (p. 59)

16. Adho Mukha Virasana with Bolster
(p. 107)

17. Supta Baddha Konasana (p. 135)

18. Savasana Side Lying (p. 149)

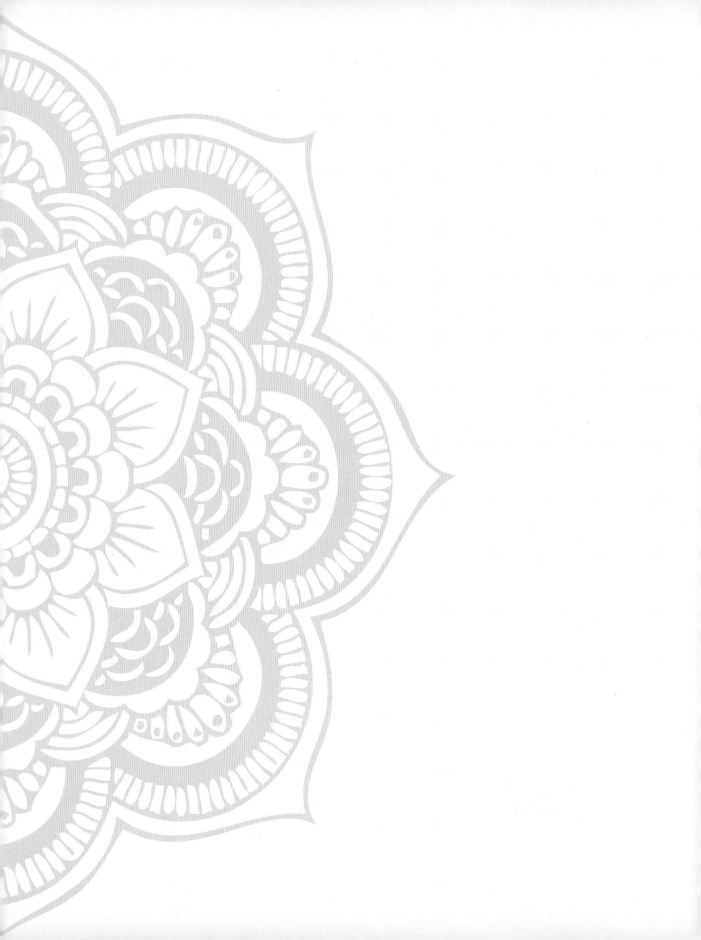

◯ Radiant
SOLAR PLEXUS CHAKRA (Manipura) मणिपूर

The solar plexus chakra, *manipura*, is like a radiant sun shining out from the base of the breastbone, where the ribs come together. This personal sunshine carries beams of empowerment, self-determination, and the ability to manifest with intention. It is the place where we feel "butterflies" before taking a risk. When we do something that requires courage and boldness (like choosing to bring a new life into the world!) we are drawing on the power of the *manipura* chakra.

This energy center is also the place from which we draw the strength to cultivate healthy boundaries. As mothers, having the clarity and self-respect to recognize and honor our individual needs is invaluable. The journey of pregnancy and motherhood often calls for putting someone else's needs first, but it's important not to lose sight of your own needs in that process. Healthy solar plexus chakra energy can help you stay true to yourself even as you nurture others. In fact, finding ways to meet your own needs is essential to being able to support your family without the fiery *manipura* chakra energy transforming into anger or resentment. Being empowered to care for yourself as well as others is nurturing not only to you but also sets a positive example for your growing family.

ॐ MANTRA

The fierce warrior goddess Durga embodies ultimate *manipura* chakra energy. Durga is the mother of the universe, and she is a potent blend of ferocity and loving-kindness. Protecting what matters takes courage and power, as demonstrated by the lion that Durga is often depicted astride, as well as the six weapons she carries in her eight hands.

While you may not have as many hands as Durga (though there will probably be plenty of times as a mother when you wish you did!), this mantra can help you embody her radiant strength.

He Ma Durga
Jai Jai Ma

Pronunciation

He = hey

Ma = mah

Durga = dure-gah

Jai = jay

For inspiration, check out Donna De Lory's album The Lover and the Beloved; the track "He Ma Durga" features this mantra.

👁 VISUALIZATION

Settle into a comfortable, reclined position, such as Savasana (p. 149). Close your eyes and bring your awareness to your solar plexus region. Envision a glowing sphere of shining golden energy radiating out from that point in all directions, like beams from the sun. Imagine its warmth and unrelenting brilliance. Feel all the compassionate strength you are capable of on behalf of yourself and your child, and allow yourself to be illuminated with that power.

○ Radiant
SOLAR PLEXUS CHAKRA (Manipura) मणिपूर

🫖 WARMING CHAI TEA

This is a delicious chai blend that is heavenly with milk and honey.

8 parts rooibos tea

½ part vanilla beans

4 parts cardamom seeds

Steep 2 teaspoons of the above mixture of tea in 1 cup hot water, with a lid on, for 15–20 minutes.

Strain and enjoy.

📖 REFLECTION & PRACTICE

One of the deepest levels of empowerment is to recognize that we never have to be victims of experience; we have the ability to choose how we show up in the world, moment by moment, breath by breath. This doesn't mean that we always have power over external events, but with practice we can control how we respond to whatever comes to us in life.

Preparing a birth plan is a wonderful expression of *manipura* chakra energy. It can be very empowering to think through your intentions, boundaries, and desires for what will be one of the most significant events of your life.

Take some time to envision your ideal birth experience. Make notes and discuss your wishes with your health care providers and your partner, or anyone who will be supporting you on the big day.

After you have done that, acknowledge that there may (and most likely will) be aspects of your baby's birth that are outside of your control. In light of that, ask yourself, what can you do to feel empowered no matter how the events of labor unfold?

⚘ Meditation for Radiant Empowerment

1. Sit in a comfortable cross-legged position, with enough blankets under you so that your knees drop down to the height of your hips or lower.

2. Close your eyes and roll them upward.

3. Sit up tall and lift from the crown of your head, lengthening your spine.

4. Bring the thumb and forefinger of your left hand together so that they make a circle; press the other three fingers together.

5. Extend and lower your left hand until the tips of your straight fingertips are resting on your left knee.

6. Press the fingers of your right hand together and raise your right arms so that your fingertips are just above the height of your head.

7. Sit in stillness for one to five minutes.

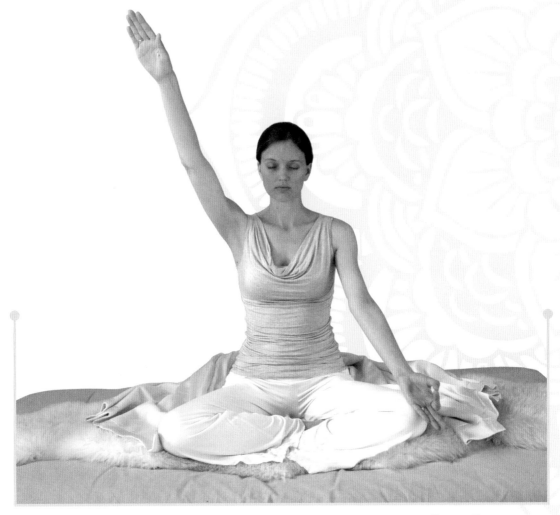

◉ Radiant Sequence 1
SOLAR PLEXUS CHAKRA (Manipura) मणिपूर

This modified sun salutation is perfect for a quick daily practice and is a great way to connect to your inner sunshine during pregnancy. Do the full sequence on one side, then repeat on the other side. Continue the full cycle as many times as desired.

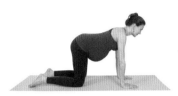

1. Hands and Knees (p. 119)

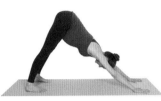

2. Adho Mukha Svanasana (p. 69)

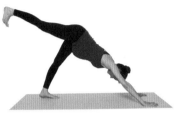

3. Eka Pada Adho Mukha Svanasana (p. 73)

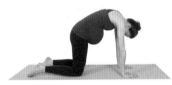

7. Cat (p. 119)

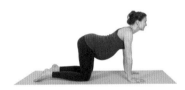

8. Cow (p. 119)

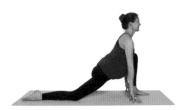

4. Lunge (p. 73)

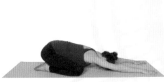

5. Adho Mukha Virasana (p. 107)

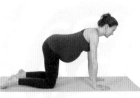

6. Hands and Knees (p. 119)

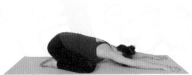

9. Sundog (p. 119)

10. Adho Mukha Virasana (p. 107)

◉ Radiant Sequence 2
SOLAR PLEXUS CHAKRA (Manipura) मणिपूर

The emphasis on standing poses in this sequence is designed to kindle the fire of your *manipura* chakra. As you move through the practice, imagine yourself like the warrior goddess Durga: courageous, radiant and strong. Realize that you are fueling a power that will be there to serve you during labor. Remember to breathe, and add in Adho Mukha Virasana as needed to create resting points.

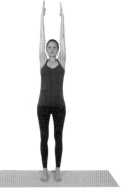

1. Tadasana (p. 15)

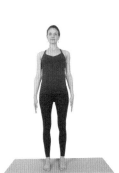

*7. Garudasana (skip in 3rd trimester) (p. 25)
(Both sides)*

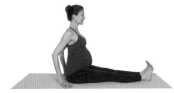

13. Dandasana (p. 77)

2. Urdhva Hastasana (p. 17)

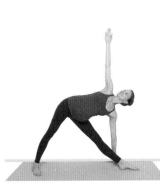

*8. Utthita Trikonasana back to wall
(p. 32) (Both sides)*

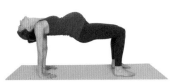

*14. Purvottanasana with head back
(p. 127)*

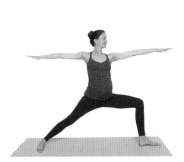

*3. Virabhadrasana II (p. 35)
(Both sides)*

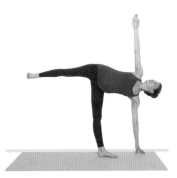

*9. Ardha Chandrasana back to wall
(p. 39) (Both sides)*

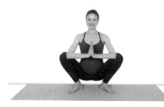

4. Parsvottanasana with Pascima
Namaskarasana Arms (p. 43) (Both sides)

5. Ardha Uttanasana (p. 51)

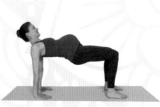

6. Virabhadrasana III (p. 55)
(Both sides)

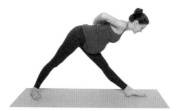

10. Squats at wall (p. 59)

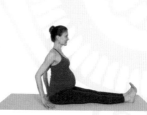

11. Dandasana (p. 77)

12. Purvottanasana (p. 127)

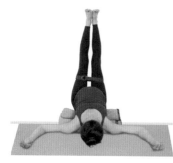

15. Viparita Karani (p. 147)

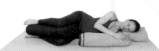

16. Side Lying Savasana (p. 149)

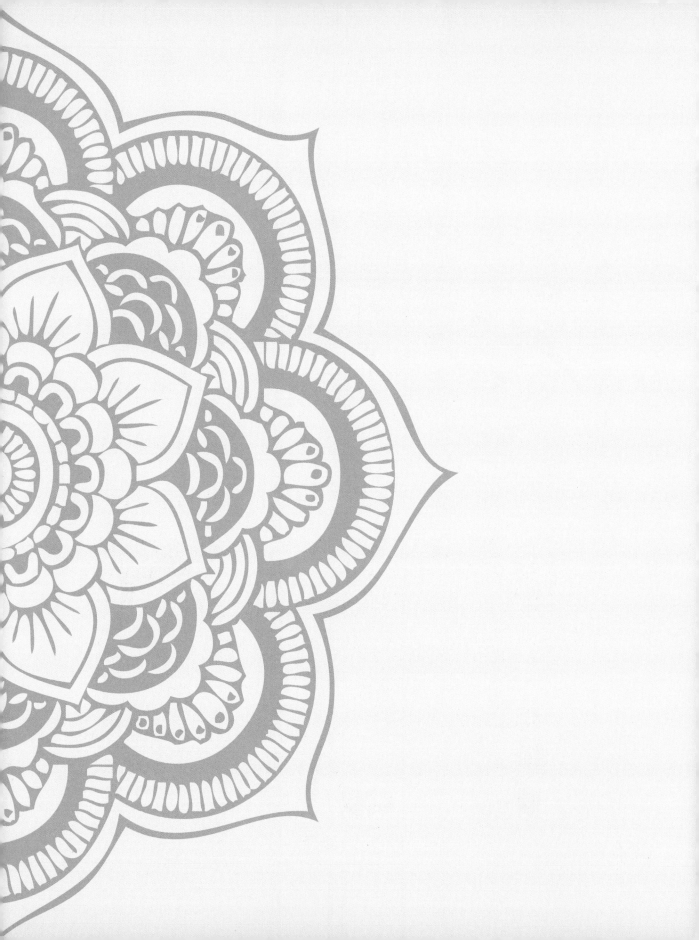

☸ Loving

HEART CHAKRA (Anahata) अनाहत

At the midway point in the chakras—with three above and three below—*anahata*, the heart chakra, is the sanctuary at the center of our being. There is a linear relationship in the expression of the chakras; as they progress from the base of the spine to the crown, each one requires the support of the ones below it. So when you are feeling grounded in your *muladhara* chakra, creative in your *svadhisthana* chakra, and radiant in your *manipura* chakra, you have a strong and confident foundation from which to experience the full beauty of the *anahata* chakra.

The heart chakra is often overflowing during pregnancy, as we are filled with feelings of tenderness and love for baby. This is a wonderful time to access and fortify the *anahata* chakra. Compassion is our true nature, and it is only when we are caught up in feelings like fear and anger (imbalances of the lower chakras) that we are blocked from experiencing ease in our hearts. When that happens, the concept of devotion can help us overcome suffering and return to the bliss of infinite love. By seeing our lives and all of our actions as an offering in service of the divine, we become free from the entanglements of our own small ego. In this way, the heart chakra is opened with full glory, and we are able to continue our journey through the higher chakras.

ॐ Mantra

The monkey god Hanuman is the ultimate servant, and as such is a beautiful reminder of how powerful *anahata* energy can be. The great Indian epic, the *Ramayana*, tells the story of how Hanuman leaped across the ocean to find Sita after she was kidnapped from her beloved Ram. This parable teaches that when we are motivated by a spirit of service, we are capable of much more than we could have ever dreamed possible.

Becoming and being a mother is the supreme experience of love and devotion. Chanting this mantra and reflecting on Hanuman's grace will remind you that seemingly impossible feats can be achieved when you are motivated by devotion. This can be powerful to remember during labor. In a spirit of service to the human being inside you, you will accomplish the creation of life— what could be more inexplicably miraculous?

Jai Jai Jai Hanuman Gosaaee

Pronunciation

Jai = jay

Hanuman = hah-noo-mahn

Gosaaee = go-sie

For inspiration, check out Krishna Das's album Breath of the Heart; the track "Baba Hanuman" features this mantra.

◉ Visualization

Settle into a comfortable, reclined position, such as Savasana (p. 149). Close your eyes and bring your awareness to the center of your chest—the energetic heart. Envision a glowing sphere of luminous emerald green energy surrounding your heart, your chest, and your upper back. Imagine the exquisite tenderness and natural grace of this infinite energy. Feel how much trust, compassion, and love you and your sweet baby are held in.

❂ Loving

HEART CHAKRA (Anahata) अनाहत

🫖 MAMA'S MILK TEA

This blend of herbs both supports healthy milk production and eases digestion for baby.

4 parts fenugreek seeds

2 parts fennel seeds

2 parts coriander seeds

2 parts oatstraw

2 parts marshmallow root

4 parts nettles

3 parts red raspberry leaf

Pour 2 teaspoons of the above mixture and 1 cup water in a small pot. Cover and simmer for 10 minutes.

Strain and enjoy. Drink 3–5 cups a day.

📖 REFLECTION & PRACTICE

Most of us experience at least occasional blockage in the *anahata* chakra. Take a moment to reflect on anything you regularly experience in life that causes you to feel constricted or hard in your heart. Are there certain obligations that trigger resentment, or certain people toward whom it is hard to feel loving? Maybe there are even moments of discomfort with your pregnancy that lead you to feel closed off from the glow of the *anahata* chakra.

For each of the things or people you identify, imagine how you could reframe your relationship from a spirit of service. How can you bring in greater compassion and devotion? Rather than feeling resentful, how can you see your actions as an open-hearted offering to something bigger? There is so much grace in experiencing life this way. The more you act from a place of service, the more loving energy you will naturally have access to. Through the path of devotion, the heart softens and the tender serenity of the *anahata* chakra infuses everything.

♣ MEDITATION FOR DEVOTION

1. Sit in a comfortable cross-legged position, with enough blankets under you so that your knees drop down to the height of your hips or lower.

2. Close your eyes and roll them upward.

3. Sit up tall and lift from the crown of your head, lengthening your spine and tucking your chin slightly.

4. Place your hands over your heart with the left hand against your chest and your right hand over it.

5. Sit quietly for 10 or more minutes, keeping the breath relaxed.

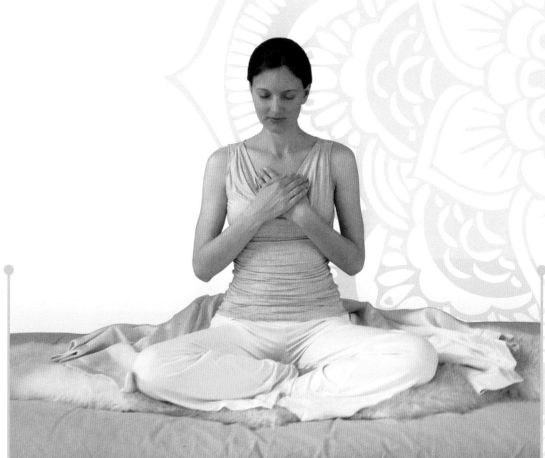

◉ Loving Sequence
HEART CHAKRA (Anahata) अनाहत

Although the chakras are part of the energetic rather than the physical anatomy, they are strongly affected by our physiology. When we collapse our shoulders and hunch our backs—which is a common tendency as our bellies grow bigger, or during breastfeeding—we close off the heart chakra. As you practice this sequence, enjoy how the feeling of opening, lifting, and broadening the chest brings energy to the *anahata* chakra. When you rest in Savasana at the end of the practice, notice the sweet tenderness you feel in your heart.

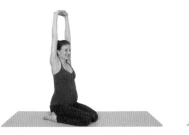

1. Virasana with Parvatasana Arms (p. 105)

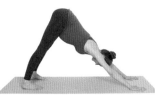

2. Adho Mukha Svanasana (p. 69)

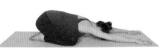

3. Adho Mukha Virasana (p. 107)

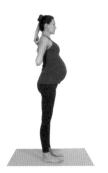

7. Gomukasana in Tadasana (p. 21) (Both sides)

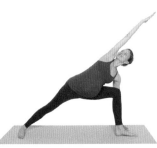

8. Parsvakonasana (p. 37) (Both sides)

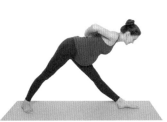

9. Parsvottanasana with Pascima Namaskarasana (p. 43) (Both sides)

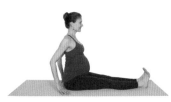

13. Dandasana (p. 77)

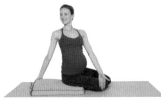

14. Bharadvajasana (p. 91) (Both sides)

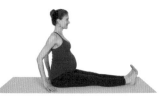

15. Dandasana (p. 77)

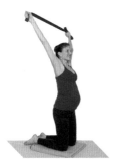

4. Kneeling Chest Opener A (p. 67)

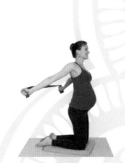

5. Kneeling Chest Opener B (p. 67)

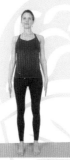

6. Tadasana (p. 15)

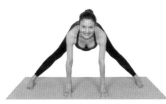

10. Prasarita Padottanasana (p. 47)

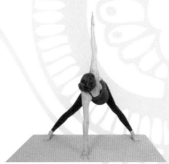

11. Prasarita Padottanasana Twist (p. 49)
(Both sides)

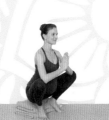

12. Squat with blankets (p. 59)

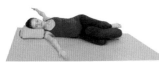

16. Side Lying Arm Circles (p. 145)
(Both sides)

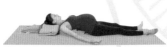

17. Pranayama Savasana (p. 155)

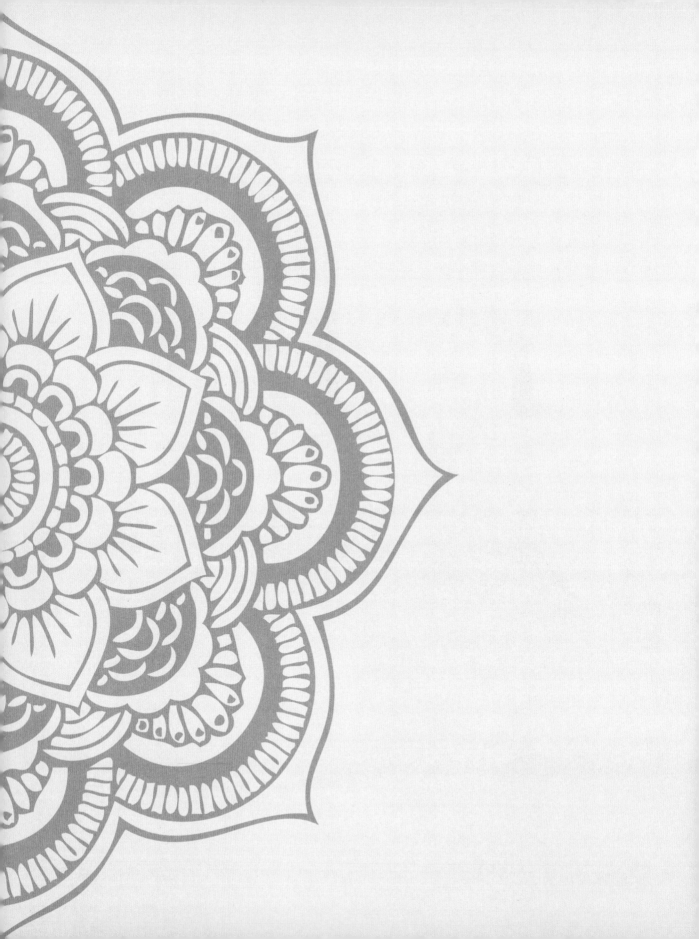

◉ Expressive
THROAT CHAKRA (Vishuddha) विशुद्ध

The throat chakra, *vishuddha*, holds our capacity for sincere, honest communication. In order to be able to speak our truth, we must first be clear in our hearts. From a balanced *anahata* chakra comes the possibility of expressing ourselves with compassion and authenticity. Being emotionally articulate is a profound skill for being able to connect deeply with others. When we understand and can speak to our experiences with clarity, we support others in being able to truly know us. This is invaluable as a parent and is a wonderful thing to be able to teach your child.

As women in Western culture, we are often indoctrinated with messages teaching us that we should say less and that our opinions or experiences are not valid. Therefore, it is not uncommon to feel blockage in the throat chakra. Working to bring balance to the *vishuddha* chakra can be incredibly liberating, as you learn to express yourself with tender honesty and fierce grace.

ॐ MANTRA

Sarasvati is the goddess of music, speech, knowledge, and wisdom. Her supreme beauty symbolizes the value and appeal of having deep understanding and being able to share it clearly. She is a gentle and lovely deity who teaches us that self-expression is a beautiful thing. Named after the mighty river that was at the heart of Indus civilization during Vedic times, Sarasvati embodies a flowing energy that characterizes healthy throat chakra energy.

Chanting in general helps bring balance and openness to the *vishuddha* chakra. This invocation to Sarasvati expresses profound respect for the goddess of expression, and helps invite her teachings into your life.

Jaya Sarasvati Jaya Jaya Devi

Pronunciation

Jaya = jay-uh

Sarasvati= sahr-uh-svah-tee

Devi = day-vee

For inspiration, check out Adam Bauer's album Shyam Lila; the track "Saraswati Devi (Jai Ma)" features this mantra.

👁 VISUALIZATION

Settle into a comfortable, reclined position, such as Supta Badha Konasana (p. 135). Close your eyes and bring your awareness to the base of your throat. Envision a glowing sphere of vibrant turquoise energy surrounding the entire throat and back of the neck. Imagine this energy melting away any blockage you may sense in this area. Feel the value of the unique truth that only you can speak, and revel in the sensation of your capacity for self-expression flowing forth unencumbered.

◉ Expressive

THROAT CHAKRA (Vishuddha) विशुद्ध

🫖 Soothing Throat ImmuniTea

This tea is healing to sore throats and is helpful when you feel a cold coming on.

2 parts marshmallow root

3 parts elder flowers

3 parts echinacea root

4 parts elder berries

Pour 2 teaspoons of the above mixture and 1 cup water in a small pot. Cover and simmer for 15–20 minutes.

Strain and enjoy. Drink throughout the day as needed.

📖 Reflection & Practice

Simple chanting is a potent tool for opening the throat chakra and finding your voice. The sacred syllable "Om" represents Universal truth. It is also spelled "aum" and when chanted is comprised of three syllables: ah-oh-m. Try chanting this simple mantra as often as you're able; it's a practice that's easy to do in the car, in the shower, or during other simple daily tasks. It's also a great way to clear energy before bed, which is a nice practice to share with older children. When you chant, breathe deeply and see if you can bring the sound all the way from your belly. Notice how repetition brings increased clarity and strength to your voice.

Vocalizing during labor can be a powerful way to move energy. Developing a chanting practice while pregnant can help build confidence in the throat chakra. This in turn prepares you to be comfortable using any and all sounds that may come to you as you labor to bring your baby into the world.

♣ Meditation for Inner Knowing

This meditation includes the silent repetition of the mantra "Sat Nam." The literal translation of this Sanskrit term is "to bow" (Nam) "to being" (Sat); the mantra is often interpreted as "Truth is my identity."

1. Sit in a comfortable cross-legged position, with enough blankets under you so that your knees drop down to the height of your hips or lower.

2. Close your eyes and roll them upward.

3. Sit up tall and lift from the crown of your head, lengthening your spine and tucking your chin slightly.

4. Fit your hands together so that the base of the left palm rests in the middle of the right palm.

5. Take a long, deep breath in, silently saying *"Sat."*

6. Exhale slowly and fully, silently saying *"Nam."*

7. Repeat for three minutes.

◉ Expressive Sequence
THROAT CHAKRA (Vishuddha) विश् द्ध

Throughout this sequence, endeavor to maintain awareness of the *vishuddha* chakra. As you engage in each pose, pay special attention to the breath, and notice any change of sensation in the throat.

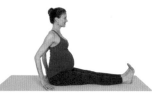

1. Toe Squat Facing Wall (p. 61)

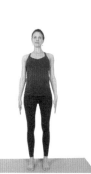

2. Tadasana (p. 15)

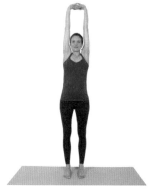

3. Baddhanguliyasana in Tadasana (p. 19)

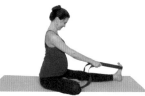

7. Dandasana (p. 77)

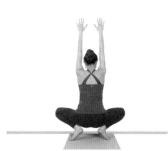

8. Maha Mudra (p. 87)
(Both sides)

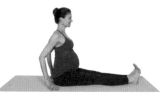

9. Dandasana (p. 77)

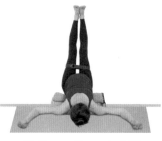

13. Viparita Karani (p. 147)

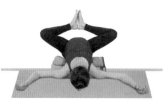

14. Viparita Karani:
Baddha Konasana Variation (p. 147)

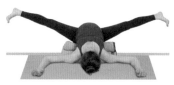

15. Viparita Karan:
Upavista Konasana Variation (p. 147)

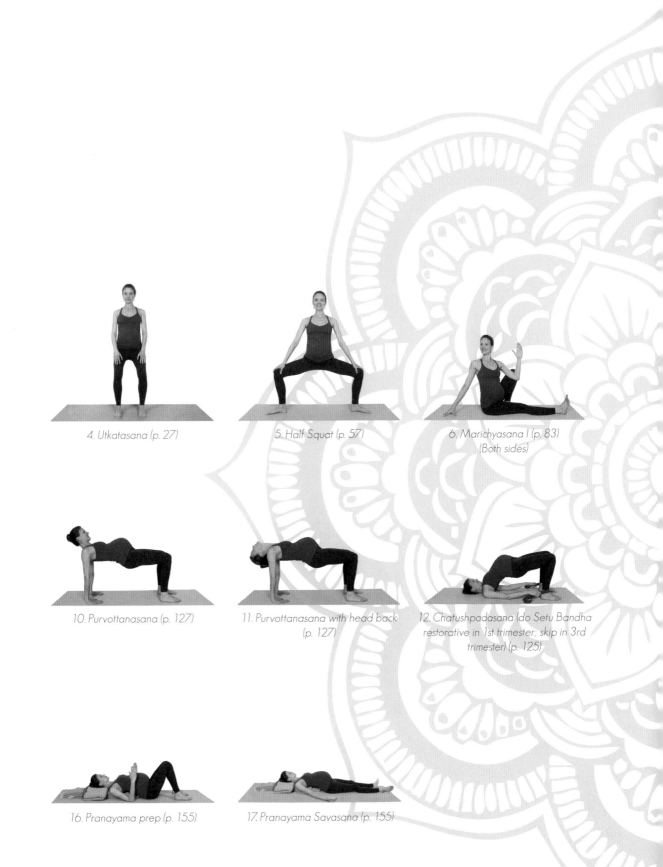

4. Utkatasana (p. 27)

5. Half Squat (p. 57)

6. Marichyasana I (p. 83)
(Both sides)

10. Purvottanasana (p. 127)

11. Purvottanasana with head back
(p. 127)

12. Chatushpadasana (do Setu Bandha
restorative in 1st trimester; skip in 3rd
trimester) (p. 125)

16. Pranayama prep (p. 155)

17. Pranayama Savasana (p. 155)

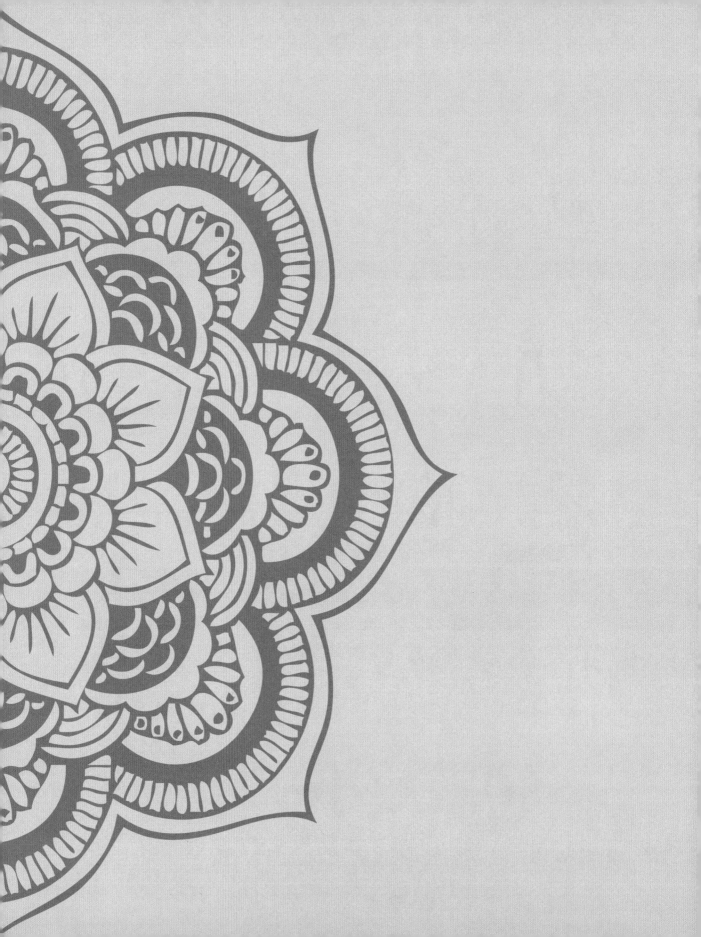

● Focused
BROW CHAKRA (Ajna) आज्ञा

Ajna, the brow chakra, connects us with our capacity for focus, clear seeing, imagination, perception, and intuition. Hormonal changes often compromise the capacity for concentration and mental focus during pregnancy and breastfeeding. When you end up at a store twenty minutes from home without your wallet, or can't find your keys anywhere, there's good reason to blame "mommy brain." This makes brow chakra work especially valuable during pregnancy. Practicing asana with attention to detail, as described in this book, is a powerful way to strengthen your capacity for single-pointed focus.

The *ajna* chakra is also related to our ability to set intention and see things through. While this can feel challenging during pregnancy, it's helpful to remember that you are actually in the process of accomplishing the most profound, important thing in the world—creating a new life! Remember that your whole being is currently engaged with incredible focus on growing your baby with unfathomable precision. If that means there's less energy left for focus of a purely mental sort, so be it—be gentle with yourself.

ॐ MANTRA

Shiva is the personification of the divine masculine, and is the deity associated with the *ajna* chakra. We all have both feminine and masculine aspects. During pregnancy, we are imbued with extra feminine energy, and attention to Shiva can bring balance. Shiva is often called the "lord of destruction." Although it may sound scary, what he actually helps break apart is the ego. This creates opening that can be permeated by divine light at the seventh and ultimate chakra.

This mantra translates as a deep bow to Shiva. In chanting it you are honoring the mental and masculine qualities within yourself. You are inviting in the divine focus that pierces through the ego and makes ultimate unity possible. Shiva also teaches us to remember that every creation of something new is preceded by destruction of something old. When things fall apart, remember to have faith in that cycle!

Hara Mahadeva
Om Nama Shivaya

Pronunciation

Hara = ha-ra

Mahadeva = mah-ha-day-vuh

Om = ohm

Nama = nam-ah

Shivaya = shee-vie-ya

For inspiration, check out Tina Malia & Shimshai's album Jaya Bhagavan; the track "Hara Hara Mahadeva" features this mantra.

◉ VISUALIZATION

Settle into a comfortable, reclined position, such as *Viparita Karani* (p. 147). Close your eyes and bring your awareness to the center of your forehead, right between the eyebrows. Envision a glowing sphere of deep indigo blue energy radiating from this point, filling your skull and the space in front of your head. Imagine this energy like a laser beam, piercing through any layers of mental doubt or confusion and bringing total clarity and single-pointed attention. Feel the unity and stillness that comes from concentrated focus.

◉ Focused

BROW CHAKRA (Ajna) आज्ञा

🫖 Peaceful Beginnings Tea

This is a calming tea, to soothe the nerves and to bring serenity and peace to your day. It can be enjoyed as needed, or used daily for deeper, more systemic benefits.

4 parts skullcap

3 parts oatstraw

2 parts spearmint

3 parts linden flower

3 parts chamomile flowers

½ part lavender

Steep 2 teaspoons of the above mixture in 1 cup of hot water for 5 minutes.

Strain and enjoy. Drink up to 3 cups a day.

📖 Reflection & Practice

Single-pointed attention on one simple thing can be a wonderful comfort measure during labor. It's hard to anticipate what you will want when the time comes, so it can be great to prepare a variety of options. Spend some time putting together a "toolkit" of things that you could focus on during labor. Your toolkit can encompass a full spectrum of visual, auditory, and kinesthetic resources. For example:

1. An image to look at. This might be a photograph of a special place or person, a beautiful painting, an image of a flower, or a drawing with geometric designs (like a mandala).

2. An object to hold. Ideally you can find something smooth or soft that is comfortable to squeeze tightly; maybe a stone from your favorite beach or a small pillow.

3. A mantra to chant. This might be a simple "Om" or maybe one of the other mantras shared in this book.

4. An encouraging phrase to think or say aloud. Reminding yourself that your body was MADE to do this can be very empowering during labor. A phrase capturing that concept in your own words can be a great anchor during labor. You could even share it with anyone who will be supporting you during the birth, and ask them to say it aloud to you during challenging moments.

5. A pose to return to. Try practicing positions from the "Postures for Labor" section of this book (starting on p. 211). Getting a good sense of the options can make it quicker to find good poses when you are actually in labor.

6. A breathing practice. Connect with the power of your breath, perhaps by using one of the pranayama sequences (beginning on p. 153). Although you won't want to use those exact practices during labor, they can be a wonderful way to deepen awareness of your breathing.

If you're able to, try collecting this toolkit a few weeks or months in advance of your due date. Then make time regularly to "visit" with each tool, infusing it with intention and meaning. The focused attention you invest now will return to serve you during labor.

⚘ MEDITATION FOR MENTAL BALANCE

1. Sit in a comfortable cross-legged position, with enough blankets under you so that your knees drop down to the height of your hips or lower.

2. Close your eyes and roll them upward.

3. Sit up tall and lift from the crown of your head, lengthening your spine and tucking your chin slightly.

4. Extend your arms out to the sides, parallel to the ground.

5. Breathing fully and deeply, begin flapping your wrists and hands; the arms should stay straight, and there is minimal movement between the wrists and shoulders.

6. Continue for three minutes.

◈ Focused Sequence

BROW CHAKRA (Ajna) आज्ञा

The balancing poses in this sequence stimulate the *ajna* chakra by calling on your capacity for single-pointed focus. The use of a *drishti*, or focused gaze, can be very useful for finding stillness in a pose, especially when you are on one leg. As you prepare to balance in Vrksasana, Virabhadrasana III, and Garudasana, choose a specific focal point in the distance. Throughout the pose, keep an unwavering focus on that spot with not only your anatomical eyes but also with the third eye that resides in your brow chakra. Notice how this brings stillness to your body, and to your entire being.

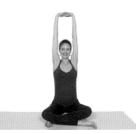

1. Svastikasana with Parvatasana Arms (p. 97)
(Both sides)

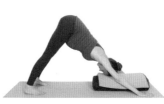

2. Adho Mukha Svanasana
with head supported (p. 69)

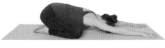

3. Adho Mukha Virasana (p. 107)

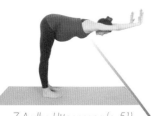

7. Ardha Uttanasana (p. 51)

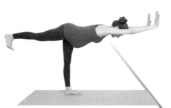

8. Virabhadrasana III (p. 55)
(Both sides)

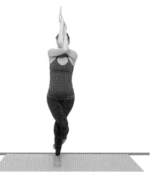

9. Garudasana (p. 25)
(Both sides)

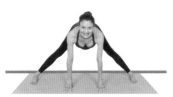

13. Prasarita Padottanasana (back to wall)
(p. 47)

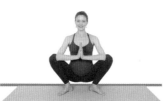

14. Squats at wall (p. 59)

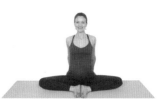

15. Baddha Konasana (p. 93)

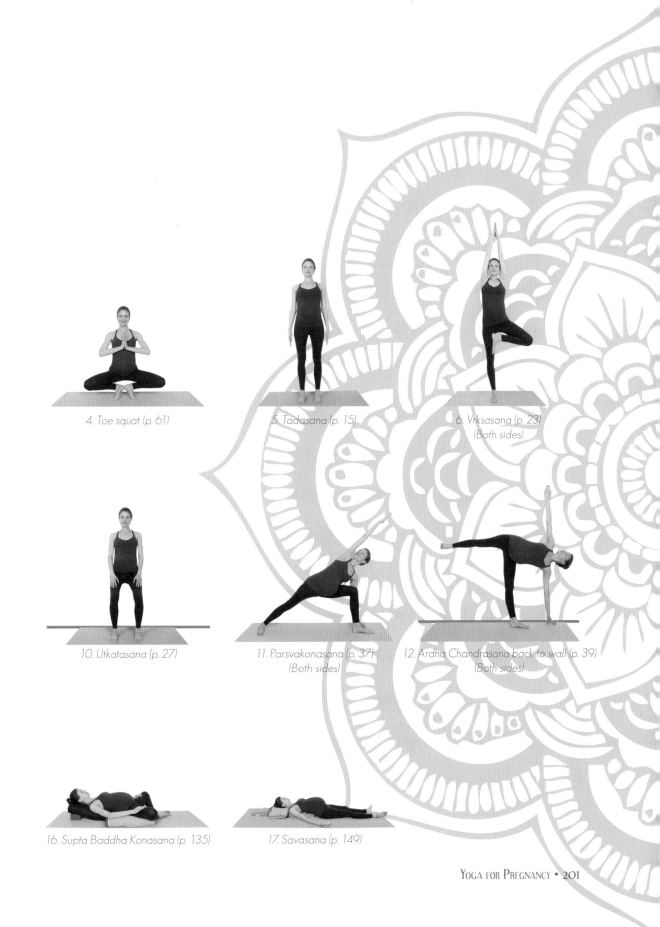

4. Toe squat (p. 61)

5. Tadasana (p. 15)

6. Vrksasana (p. 23)
(Both sides)

10. Utkatasana (p. 27)

11. Parsvakonasana (p. 37)
(Both sides)

12. Ardha Chandrasana back to wall (p. 39)
(Both sides)

16. Supta Baddha Konasana (p. 135)

17. Savasana (p. 149)

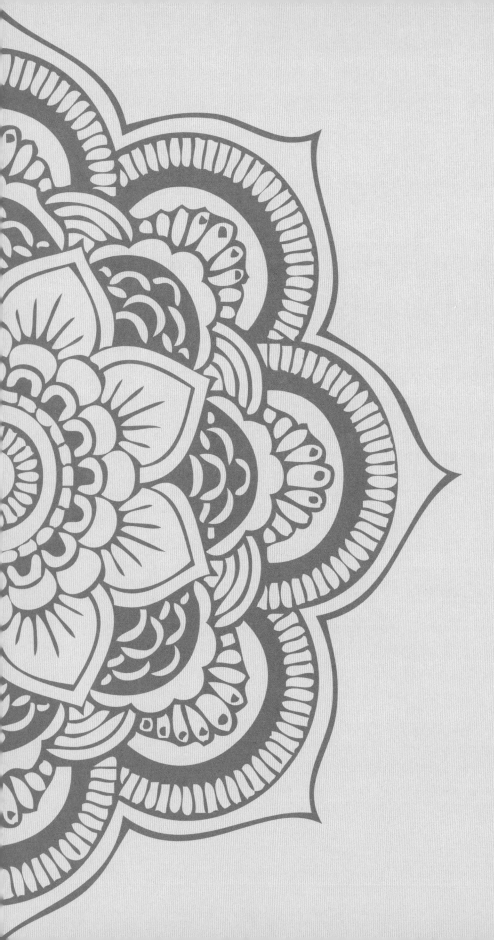

◉ Divine

CROWN CHAKRA (Sahasrara) सहसरार

The seventh and final chakra, the *sahasrara*, or crown, chakra is a portal to divine transcendence. When we have learned the lessons of the other six chakras, we are ready to taste the bliss of sacred connection with infinity. The transcendence of the crown chakra isn't about escaping our bodies or leaving reality behind. Rather, it is an experience of overcoming the illusion of separateness. During the majority of our waking life, most of us suffer from the misperception that we are isolated beings, and we often feel hopelessly overwhelmed by our ideas about what we are supposed to be accomplishing. When we are stuck in thinking that it is up to us to make things happen, to push the proverbial boulder up the hill, all alone, we are bound to suffer.

The *sahasrara* chakra allows us to remember that we are not alone; we are, in fact, held afloat in a beautiful river of divine light that flows through all of existence. Our most important work in life is to remember this truth. When we are balanced and clear, we become channels for divinity, serving the world and the people around us from a place of sacred connection. This often requires releasing attachment to our ideas about what is supposed to be happening. From humble surrender comes the ability to access a higher power, as we learn to flow with grace through even the rapids of life.

These crown chakra lessons are especially potent as you prepare to dive into motherhood. There will inevitably be moments when it feels impossible to juggle all the demands of your life *and* meet your baby's needs. When those moments come, draw on these *sahasrara* practices and remember that there is a divine intelligence at work, and you are completely supported. All will be well.

ॐ Mantra

This mantra to the universal divine mother is deeply inspiring to practice while pregnant. It is a reminder that you are supported by an infinitely nurturing feminine principle, and that you are also an embodiment of this divinity.

Omkar Guru Ma Omkar Jai Jai Ma

Pronunciation

Omkar = ohm-car

Guru = goo-roo

Ma = mah

Jai = jay

For inspiration, check out Wah!'s album Savasana; the track "Omkar Guru Ma" features this mantra.

👁 Visualization

Settle into a comfortable, reclined position, such as Savasana (p. 149). Close your eyes and bring your awareness to the crown of your head. Envision a glowing sphere of luminous violet energy surrounding this point. Imagine this energy expanding outward with infinite radiance. Feel the divinity within you and surrounding you; know that this sacred bliss is always present and available to you when you become still enough to experience it.

◉ Divine

CROWN CHAKRA (Sahasrara) सहस्रार

🫖 BLOSSOMING MAMA BLEND

This is a fantastic light floral tea that tastes great and is soothing to the system.

4 parts elder flowers

4 parts linden flowers

4 parts lemon verbena

2 parts marshmallow root

Steep 2 teaspoons of the above mixture in 1 cup hot water for at least 10 to 20 minutes.

Strain and enjoy. Drink up to 3 cups a day hot or cold. This is a delicious iced tea in the warmer months to refresh and renew.

📖 REFLECTION AND PRACTICE

The following practice is inspired by a teaching from Swami Radha, a German-born yogini who founded the Yasodhara Ashram in British Columbia. It is a powerful tool for activating *sahasrara* energy.

Divine Light Invocation

I am created by Divine Light.

I am sustained by Divine Light.

I am protected by Divine Light.

I am surrounded by Divine Light.

I am ever growing into Divine Light.

1. Stand in Tadasana (p. 15) with your eyes closed. Inhale slowly, silently saying the invocation above. As you inhale, raise your arms out to the side and up overheard, imagining yourself being filled with divine light.
2. Exhale and lower your arms down in front of you, bringing them to rest on your belly. Imagine the light filling you from the crown of your head down to your toes.
3. Repeat, and this time as you exhale, bring your arms out in front of you, as though you are holding a giant beach ball. Imagine the spherical space between your arms being filled with a pool of divine light.
4. Envision the sweet, pure soul of your baby being held in that pool of light. Keeping your arms steady, inhale and repeat the invocation again, this time replacing the "I" pronoun with "you" so that you are saying it to your baby.
5. As you exhale, bring your hands to your belly, drawing that whole pool of divine light into the being who is growing inside you.

⚜ Meditation for Infinite Connection

1. Sit in a comfortable cross-legged position, with enough blankets under you so that your knees drop down to the height of your hips or lower.

2. Close your eyes and roll them upward.

3. Sit up tall and lift from the crown of your head, lengthening your spine and tucking your chin slightly.

4. Cup your hands together in front of your heart, a few inches from your chest.

5. Sit quietly for 10 or more minutes, keeping the breath relaxed.

◉ Divine Sequence
CROWN CHAKRA (Sahasrara) सहस्रार

This is a blissful restorative sequence, wonderful for anytime you feel tired or in need of some divine nurturing. You will notice that it is a short sequence; this is because all but pose #3 should be enjoyed for 10–15 minutes each. As you practice, let yourself completely relax into each pose. Make sure you are in a quiet space that is a comfortable temperature. If you notice at any point that you are feeling anything less than completely at ease, try making adjustments to your position or props.

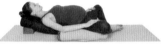

1. Supta Baddha Konasana (p. 135)

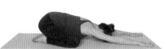

2. Adho Mukha Virasana (p. 107)

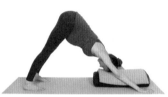

3. Adho Mukha Svanasana head supported (p. 69)

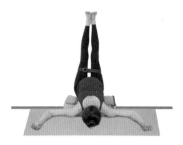

7. Viparita Karani (p. 147)

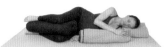

8. Side Lying Savasana (p. 149)

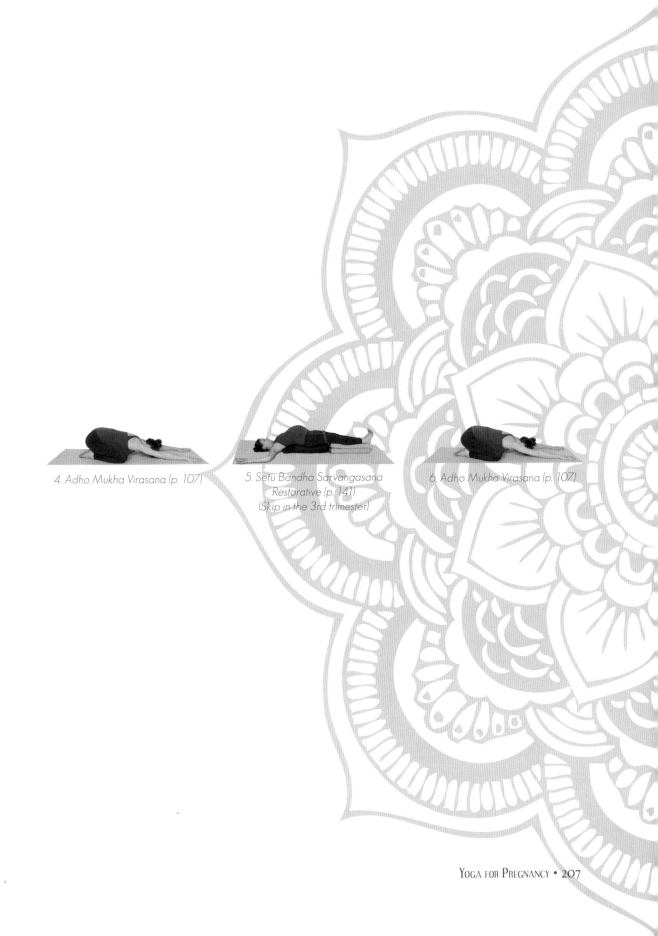

4. Adho Mukha Virasana (p. 107)

5. Setu Bandha Sarvangasana
Restorative (p. 141)
(Skip in the 3rd trimester)

6. Adho Mukha Virasana (p. 107)

Full Chakra Meditation

Once you have practiced visualizing each chakra individually, it is profound to experience them sequentially, in relationship to one another. You can do this as a stand-alone practice, or you can incorporate it into Savasana following any asana sequence.

Settle into a comfortable, reclined position, such as Savasana. Close your eyes and bring your awareness to the bottom of your torso. Envision a glowing sphere of deep red energy surrounding the base of your spine, your perineum, and your pubic bone. Imagine this energy spreading through your legs like roots of a tree, stabilizing you and connecting you with the earth. Feel how the ground is supporting you and your baby unconditionally; let yourself be heavy, melting into gravity completely.

From this vibrant energy in the root chakra, visualize a column of white light growing up from the perineum and into the belly. Envision this column of light growing into a glowing sphere of vibrant orange energy surrounding your lower abdomen and low back. Imagine this energy holding your precious baby in its light. Feel your own vast capacity for creativity and sustenance; let yourself silently hum with the glow of fertility and sensuality.

Continuing to feel bright and strong in your first two chakras, visualize that column of white light growing up from the perineum, through the belly, and into the solar plexus. Envision the column of light growing into a glowing sphere of shining golden energy radiating out from your solar plexus in all directions, like beams from the sun. Imagine its warmth and unrelenting brilliance. Feel all the compassionate strength you are capable of on behalf of yourself and your child, and let yourself be lit up with that power.

Continuing to feel bright and strong in your first three chakras, visualize that column of white light growing up from the perineum, through the belly, through the solar plexus, and into the center of your chest. Envision the column of light growing into a glowing sphere of luminous emerald green energy surrounding your heart, your chest, and your upper back. Imagine the exquisite tenderness and natural grace of this infinite energy. Feel how much trust, compassion, and love you and your sweet baby are held in.

Continuing to feel bright and strong in your first four chakras, visualize that column of white light growing up from the perineum, through the belly, through the solar plexus, through the center of your chest, and into your throat. Envision the column of light growing into a glowing sphere of vibrant turquoise energy surrounding the entire throat and back of the neck. Imagine this energy melting away any blockage you may sense in this area. Feel the value of the unique truth that only you can speak, and revel in the sensation of your capacity for self-expression flowing forth unencumbered.

Continuing to feel bright and strong in your first five chakras, visualize that column of white light growing up from the perineum, through the belly, through the solar plexus, through the center of your chest, through your throat, and into the third eye point at the center of your forehead. Envision the column of light growing into a glowing sphere of deep indigo blue energy radiating from this point, filling your skull and the space in front of your head. Imagine this energy like a laser beam, piercing through any layers of mental doubt or confusion and bringing total clarity and single-pointed attention. Feel the unity and stillness that comes from concentrated focus.

Continuing to feel bright and strong in your first six chakras, visualize that column of white light growing up from the perineum, through the belly, through the solar plexus, through the center of your chest, through your throat, through your third eye, and into the crown of your head. Envision the column of light growing into a glowing sphere of luminous violet energy surrounding the top of your head. Imagine this energy expanding outward with infinite radiance. Feel the divinity within you and surrounding you; know that this sacred bliss is always present and available to you when you become still enough to experience it.

To finish, imagine a white light pouring through the crown of your head and infusing your entire body with vitality and healing. Let yourself be completely replenished and nourished by the universal life force.

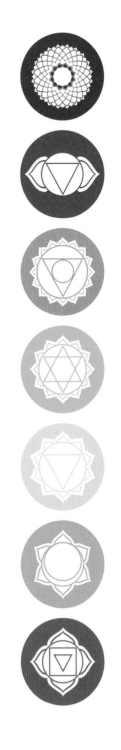

Postures
for
Labor

BEING CREATIVE with your positions during labor can bring ease and help the birth progress smoothly. This section features a variety of poses to do on your own or with anyone who will support you during your labor. Consider practicing them ahead of time and keeping this book as a handy reference during labor.

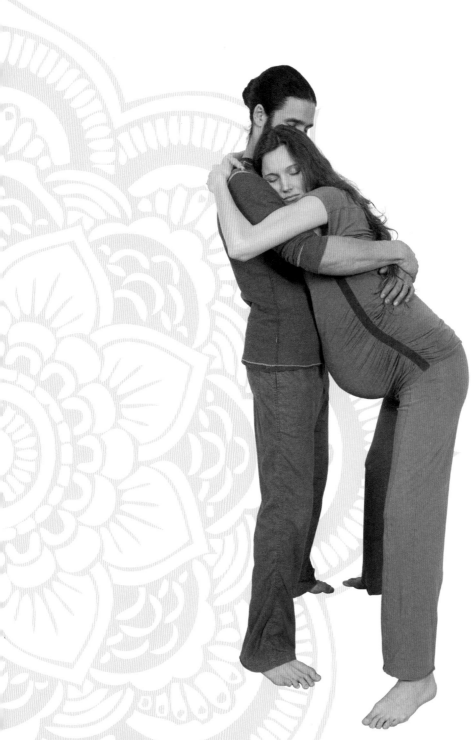

Slow Dancing

Slow dancing with your partner is a great way to gently keep your hips moving and connect with each other.

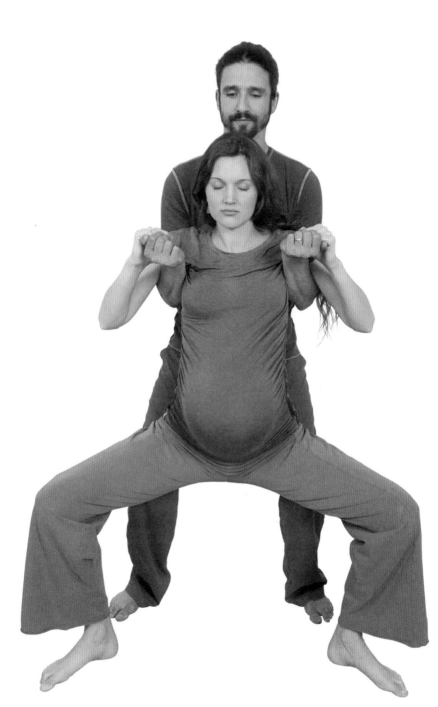

Supported Standing Squat

Moving around and changing positions is invaluable during labor. This is a helpful standing squat position where your partner is supporting your weight. Try this way of squatting during a contraction and then come to "Standing with Emotional Support," "Slow Dancing," or rest your head on a high comfortable surface in between contractions.

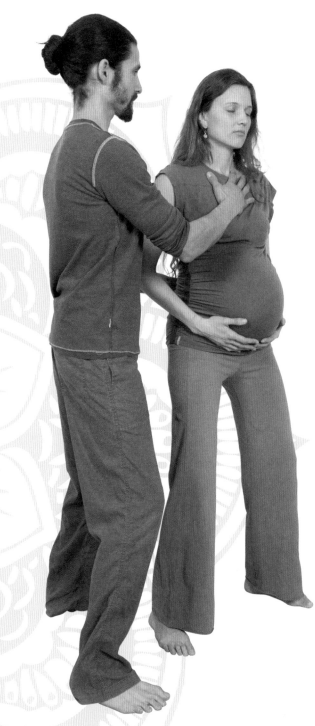

Standing with Emotional Support

Have a support person place a hand of support on your shoulder or chest in between contractions and focus on connecting with you emotionally. More physical support can be given when needed.

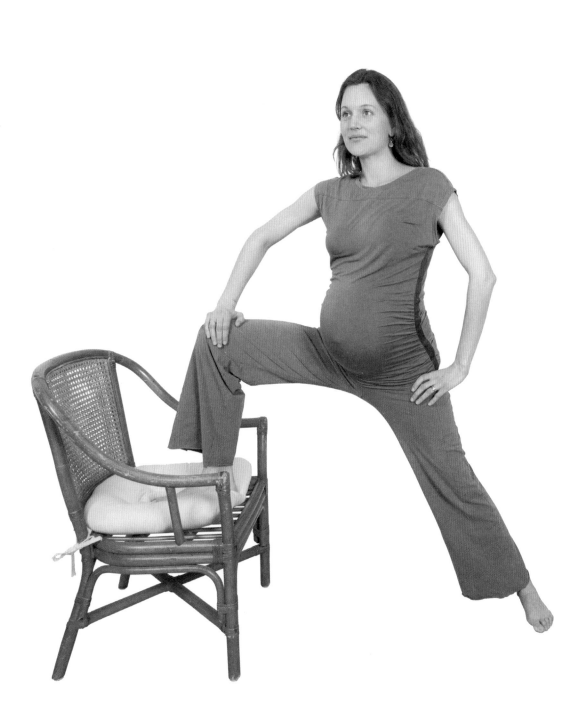

SIDE LUNGE

This can be very helpful in prelabor and also during labor for getting baby to descend deeper into the birth canal.

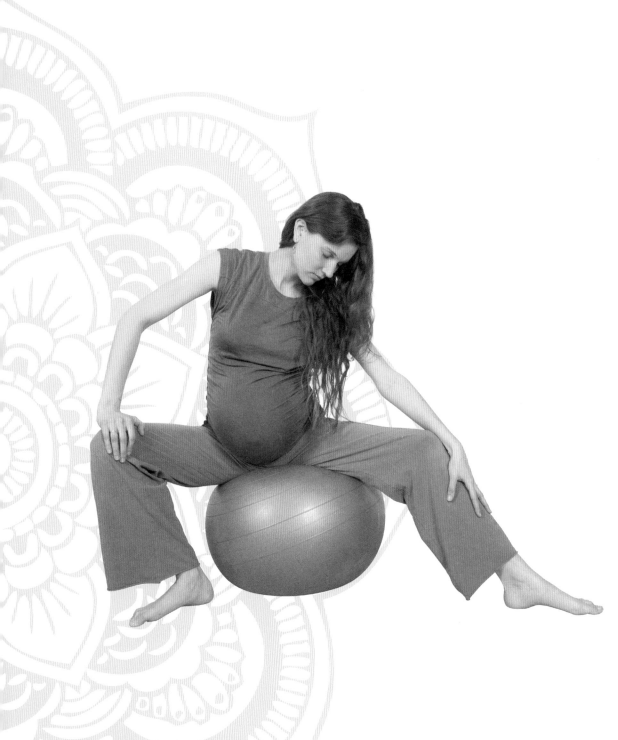

Yoga Ball Hip Circles

The birth ball is a fantastic prop to have available during labor. This picture demonstrates doing hip circles on the ball. Moving the hips in this way creates openings in the pelvic bones for baby to wiggle further down into the birth canal.

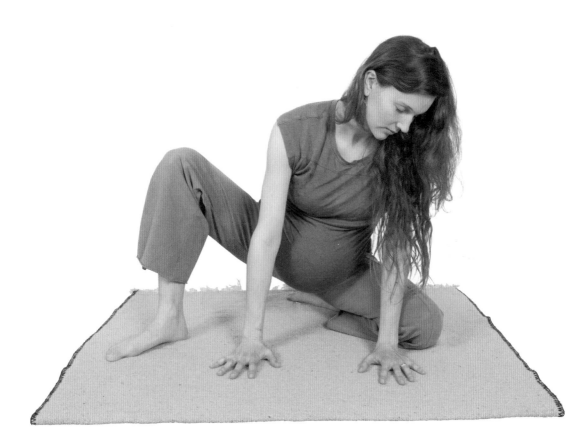

Side Lunge Squat

Combining different postures after every few contractions can help baby find new space to wiggle down into. This is another posture to add to opening the hips when you are on the floor. Try this for a few contractions on each side, resting in between in a Supported Child's Pose variation.

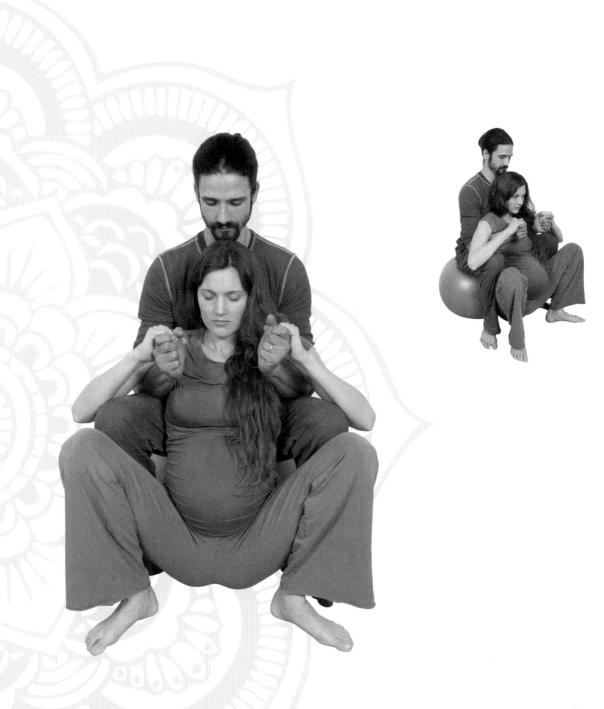

Supported Squat with Partner

Your partner can utilize the birth ball too. Notice how Noah's arms are supporting Megan's underarms. This gives maximum support as she is able to freely dangle. This can also be done with the partner/support person sitting on a chair or yoga ball.

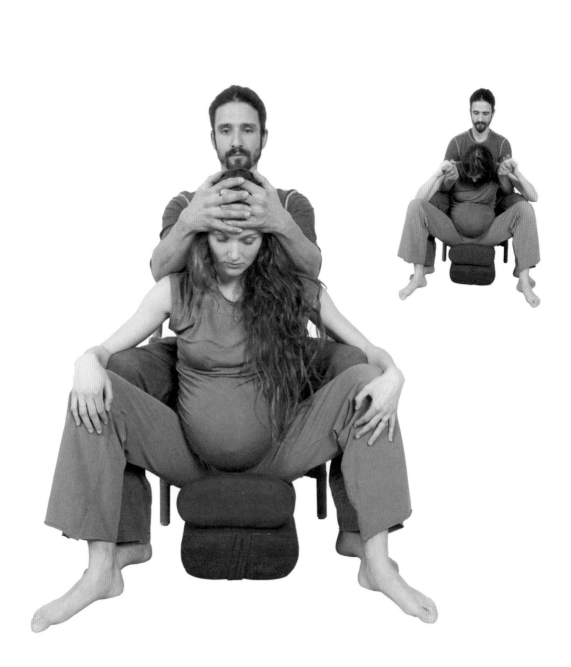

Seated Supported Squat with Partner

Another way to squat is while sitting on some support like the two bolsters in this photo. A small stool or folded blankets could also work. The same actions apply as in the supported squat. In this position the partner can hold either the hands or support the head.

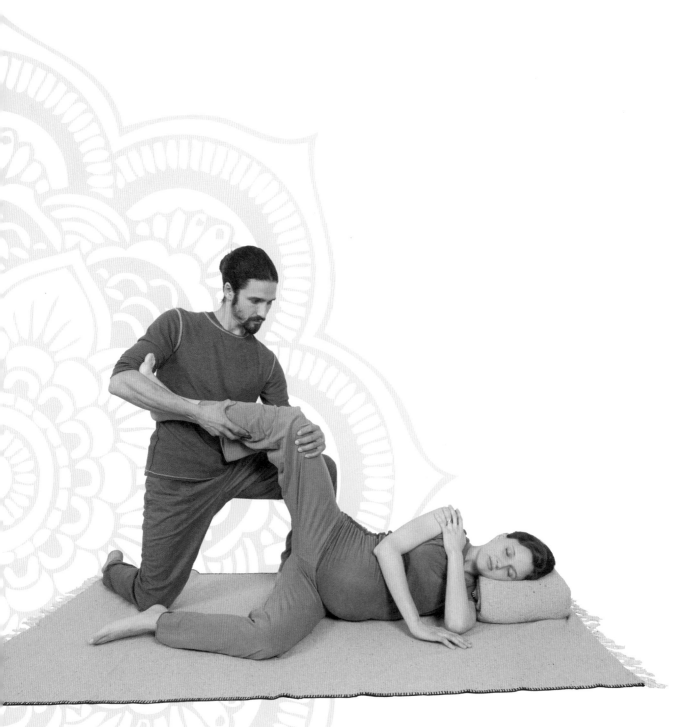

SIDE LYING LEG SUPPORTED

Side lying in this way can be a great position for pushing. In side lying you don't have to hold your body up at all and your partner or doula can support your leg and press into your feet to open the hips wider. It is helpful during pushing to take the knee all the way in toward the chest. Pushing and birthing in this antigravity position can also prevent or lessen tearing.

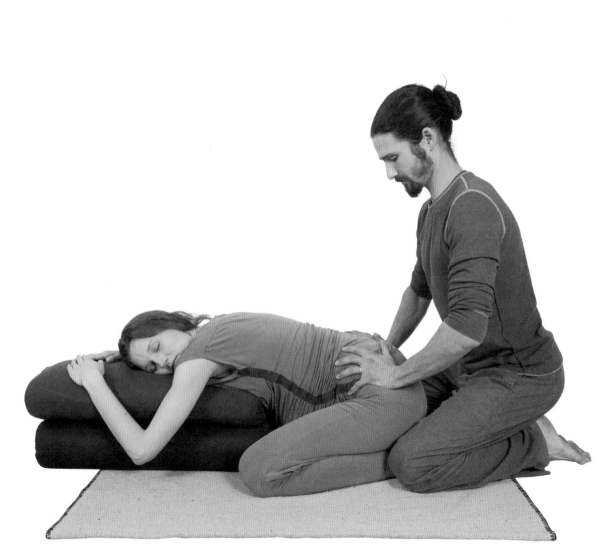

Double Hip Squeeze

Having someone squeeze the tops of the pelvic bones in toward one another in labor can give major relief when there is low back pain. It broadens the hips and relieves some of the pressure of baby pressing on the bones.

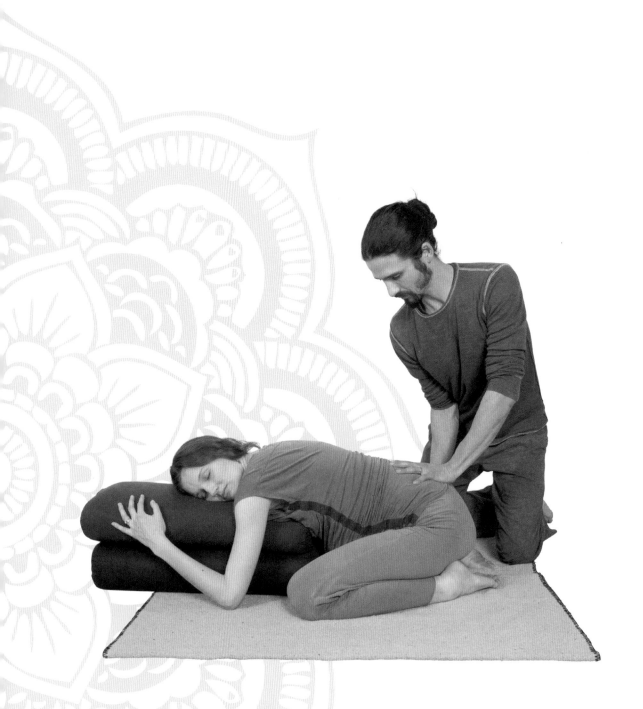

Sacral Counter Pressure

With the base of the palm, press right on the sacral bone. This can be done in many of these postures and it can take a lot of pain out of the low back during a contraction.

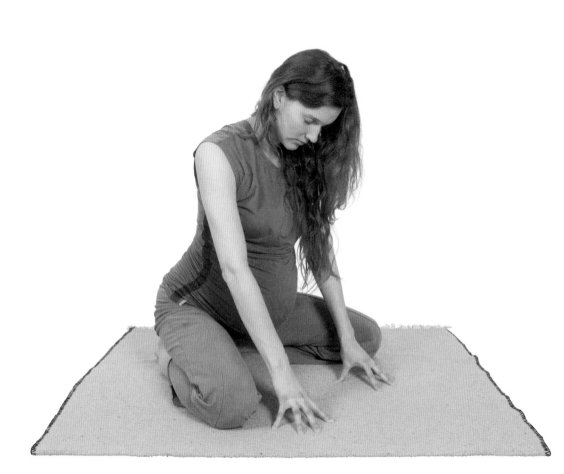

Upright Child's Pose

During the actual contractions this pose can be helpful to encourage the baby to move downward more quickly. Between contractions, rest in a Supported Child's Pose variation.

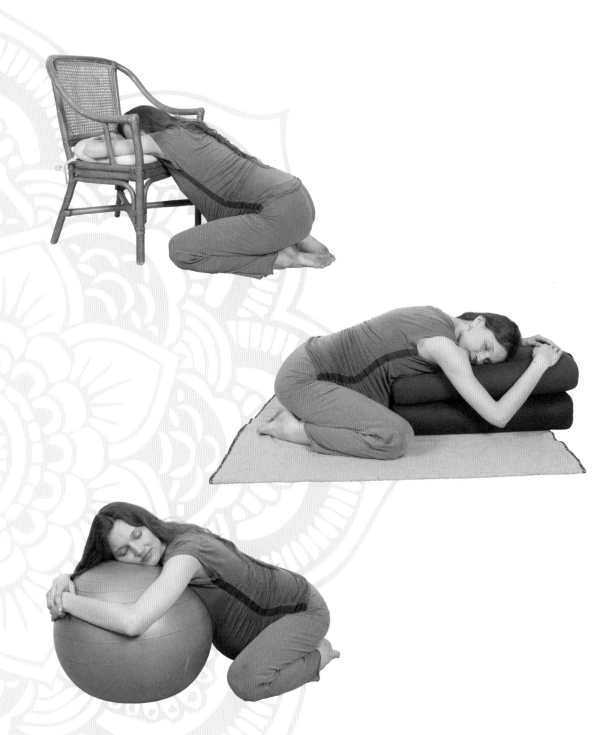

Supported Child's Pose

This pose, as well as all forward bend postures, encourages baby's spine to rotate toward the floor due to gravity. The baby's spine is heavier than his or her belly. This is an advantageous position for birthing, especially if back pain is involved due to the baby being rotated occiput posterior. In this posture, the hips are also very open and your head can rest. It is an excellent birthing position! You can use a chair, bolsters, or a yoga ball for support.

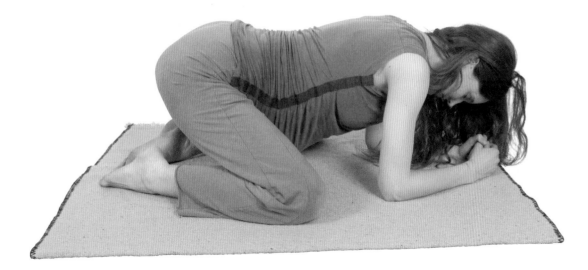

Hands and Knees

This pose is invaluable during labor and during the crowning time. Like the Supported Child's Pose variations, the weight of the baby moves a bit away from your low back and encourages a good occiput anterior position. When there is a stack of pillows under the chest, the mother can rest in between the contractions.

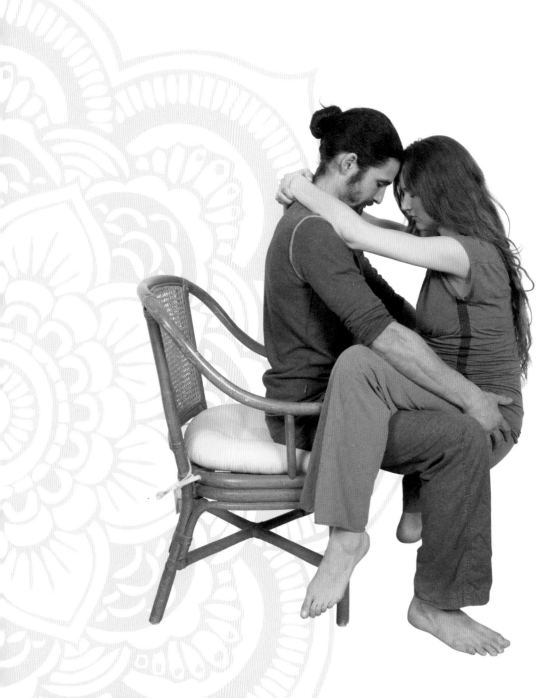

Lap Squat

This is an excellent supportive posture that helps baby descend. You can rest your head on your partner in between contractions.

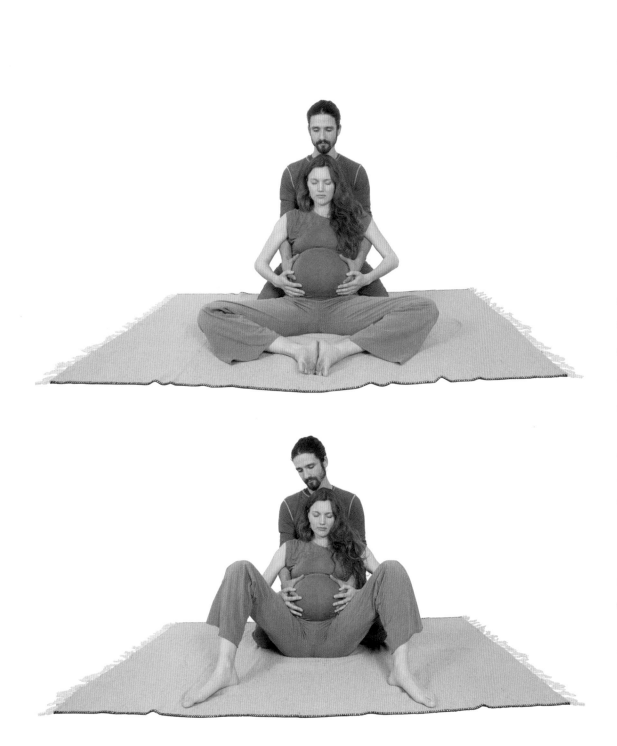

Seated Support

This is a fantastic posture for birthing the baby. By leaning back on your partner and keeping the feet wide, you allow baby to come through more easily.

Postpartum Poses and Practices

This section includes postpartum practices for baby, for you and baby together, and for you on your own.

While there are many yoga poses that can be included in a safe, healthy postpartum practice, this section features a handful of the ones that are especially valuable during this time of recovery and rebuilding.

It is important to wait at least 6–8 weeks after delivery before resuming your practice. Do not do any asanas while there is postpartum bleeding. In cases of caesarean section, wait until the incision has fully healed before practicing these poses (at least 8 weeks).

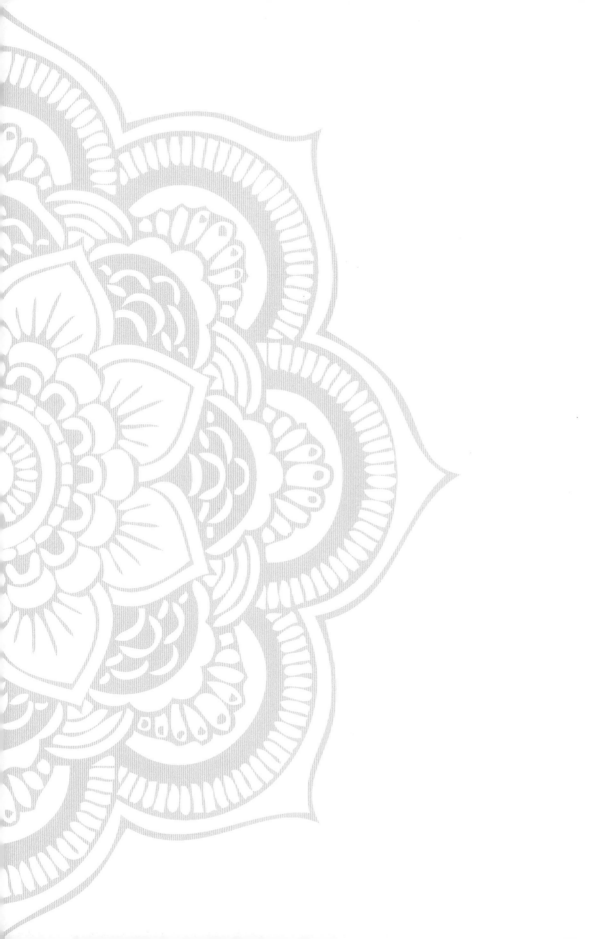

Yoga for Baby

Note: Since the baby pictured is a boy (Megan's son Robin Wilder), we have opted to use masculine pronouns. Please translate to "she" and "her" if your baby is a girl.

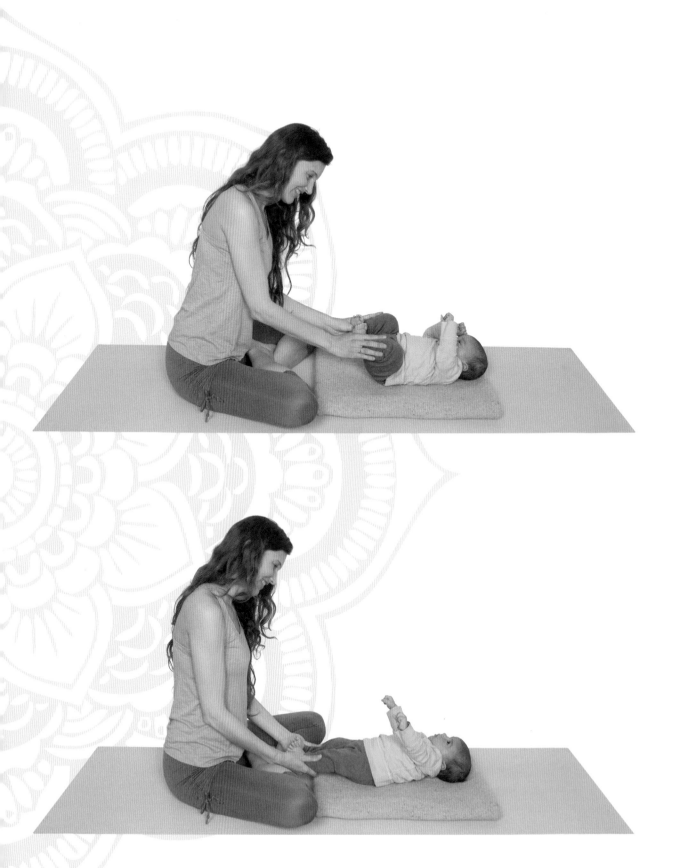

Pavanamuktasana
Wind Relieving Pose

This pose is great for "wind relieving" if baby is fussy due to an upset tummy. Assisting baby's legs to move in this way can allow the wind to pass.

Lie baby down on a blanket on the floor and bend knees into his chest and then straighten his legs. You can repeat this for as long as baby is enjoying it. You can also take knees even closer into baby's chest, lifting his buns up into the air. Many babies really like this. Also try wiggling baby side to side gently when you straighten his legs.

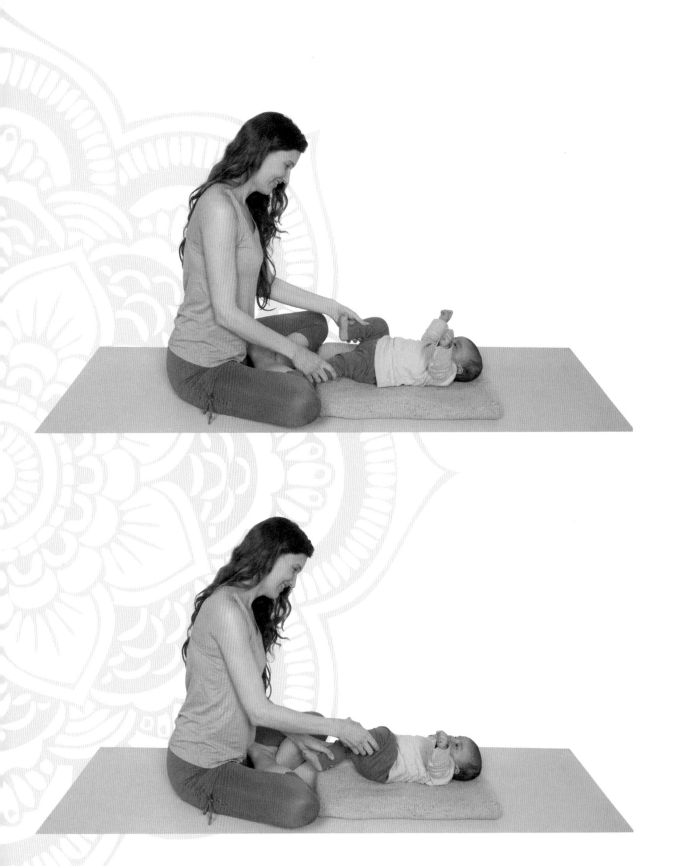

Bicycle Legs

This pose can help stimulate baby's digestive tract if there is an upset tummy, and it is a great way to engage and bond with your baby.

Lie baby down on the floor on a blanket. Hold on to baby's lower legs and take one knee into the chest while you straighten the opposite leg. Baby's legs look like he is riding a bicycle.

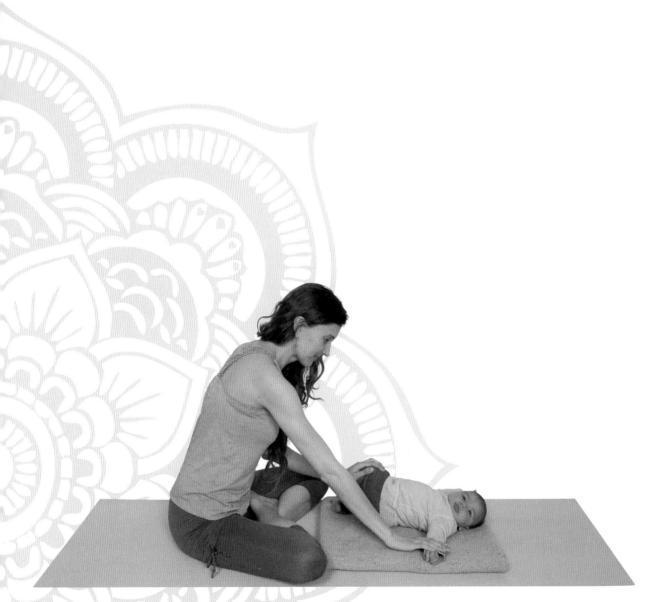

Baby Twist

Doing baby twists can be another aid to baby if colic or fussiness is due to an upset tummy.

1. With one of your hands, bend baby's knees into his chest and take his legs up toward his right armpit and down toward the floor.
2. With your other hand, stretch baby's left arm out to the left in line with his shoulder.
3. Be mindful to notice where his little body is feeling a stretch and stay there, not going beyond that point.
4. Repeat on the second side.
5. You can repeat this quite a few times on each side until baby is ready for something new.

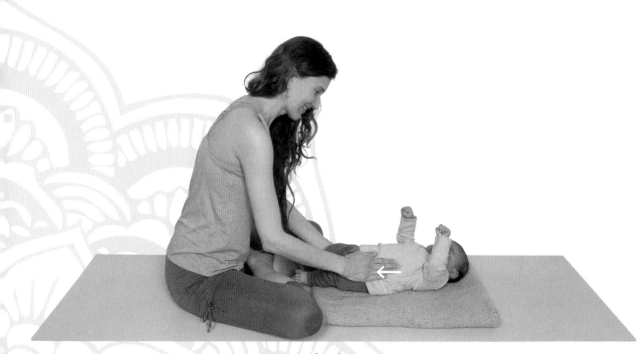

Step 1

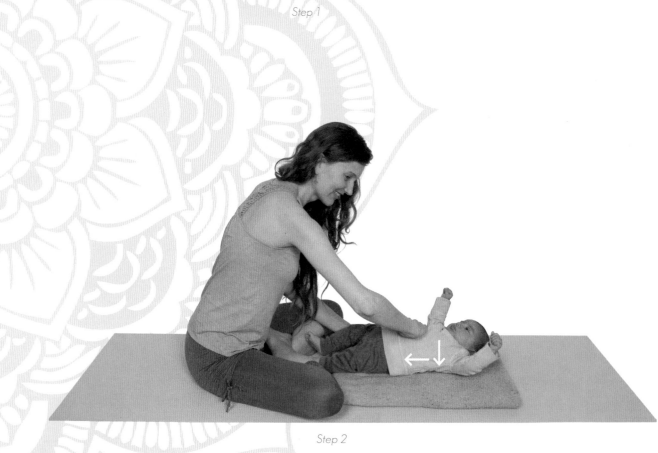

Step 2

I Love You Baby Massage

If baby is upset, you can try giving his tummy this little massage to stimulate the large intestine to empty. Your fingers are tracing along baby's large intestine, making the shapes of I, L, and U. The instructions for this massage are in relation to baby's right and left, not the person giving the massage.

1. Lie baby down on a blanket on the floor. Sit in front of your baby. Take your hand and gently stroke baby's tummy down from his top left side of the belly to his bottom left side. This is the "I" shape of the massage. Do this action a few times (see Step 1).

2. Next take your hand and massage baby from his right upper belly to his left upper belly and then down to the left lower belly again like above in the "I" shape. This shape is like an upside down "L," standing for Love in the "I Love You" massage. Repeat this L shape a few times (see Step 2).

3. Finally, take your hand and massage from baby's lower right belly up to the upper right belly, then over to his left upper belly and again down to his left lower belly. This action is like an upside down "U," standing for YOU in the "I Love You" massage. Repeat this U shape a few times (see Step 3).

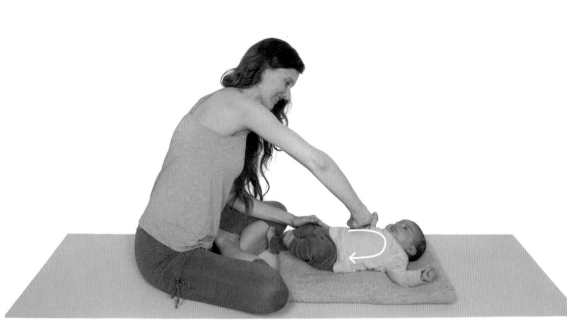

Step 3

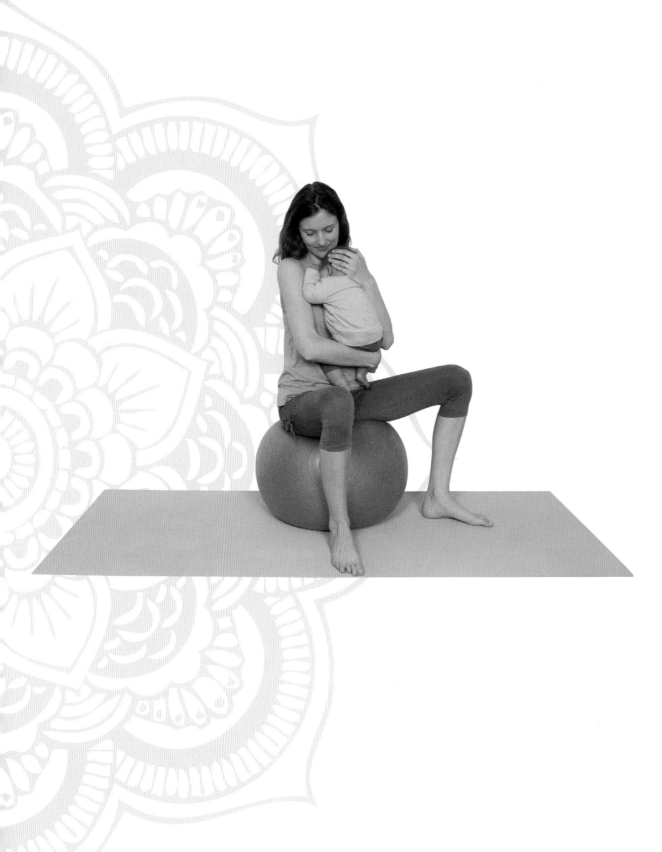

Yoga Ball Bounce

All babies love rhythmic movement. This is a great way to get your baby to sleep. You can also try this on the edge of a bed, if you do not have a yoga ball (a yoga ball is preferable to a bed though, because you can get a bigger bounce). It is great leg and core strengthening for you, too.

1. Sit on a yoga ball with your feet wide apart for balance. With one hand, support baby's head and lean his little body into your chest.
2. With your other hand, support baby under his little buns.
3. Then bounce to a rhythm. It is great to add some music that is calming with a steady beat. Babies love a heartbeat rhythm; it is comforting to them.
4. You can also try bouncing or walking to a rhythm, holding baby in a baby carrier.

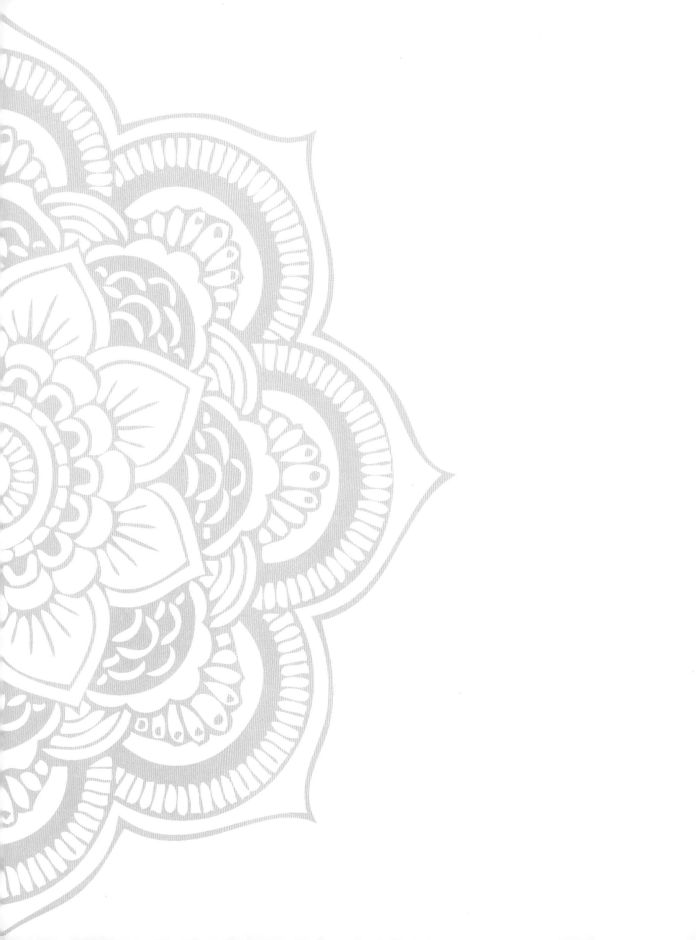

Yoga with Baby

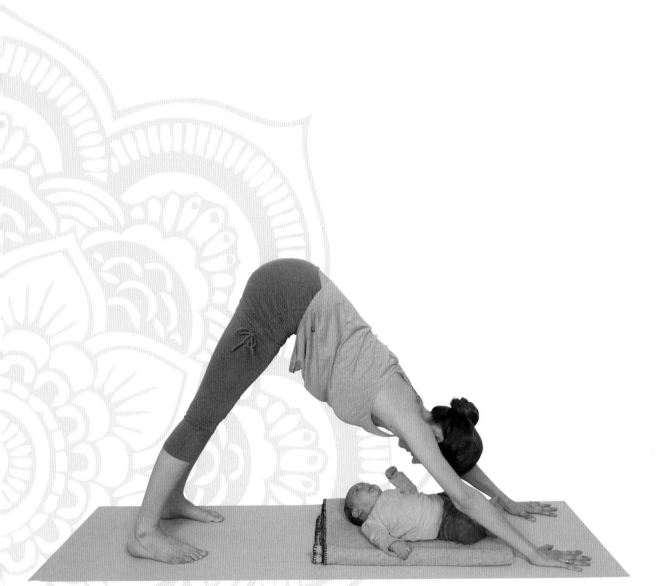

Adho Mukha Svanasana with Baby

Downward Facing Dog Pose with Baby

In this pose, you can activate and lengthen your whole body while still being attentive to your little baby. Older babies really like to pull your hair in the pose—watch out!

COMING INTO THE POSE

1. Place a blanket on the floor on your sticky mat.
2. Place baby on the blanket with his feet pointing toward the end edge of your sticky mat.
3. Come to your hands and knees with your hands in front of the blanket.
4. Slide your knees two inches back from the hips.
5. Spread your fingers wide and press the mounds of the pointer fingers firmly down.
6. Rotate the upper arms out and take your shoulders away from the ears.
7. Take the sternum bone forward.
8. Look forward.
9. Keeping the chest and head forward, turn the toes under.
10. Take a deep inhalation and exhale to lift the hips up.
11. Release your head and neck.

ENGAGING ACTIONS

1. Keep rotating the upper arms out and press into the mounds of the fingers.
2. Inhale; lift the sitting bones and outer hips higher.
3. Lift up and out of the shoulders.
4. Exhale; keep the hips lifted; press the front of the thighs back toward the back of the thighs; press the inner thighs back so the legs are super firm.
5. If you can keep your hips fully lifted, press the heels toward the floor.
6. Soften your eyes, relax your face, and let the breath flow freely.

Stay for 5–10 breaths.

COMING OUT OF THE POSE:

1. Come back to hands and knees.
2. Lower into Adho Mukha Virasana (p. 107) and rest for a few breaths.

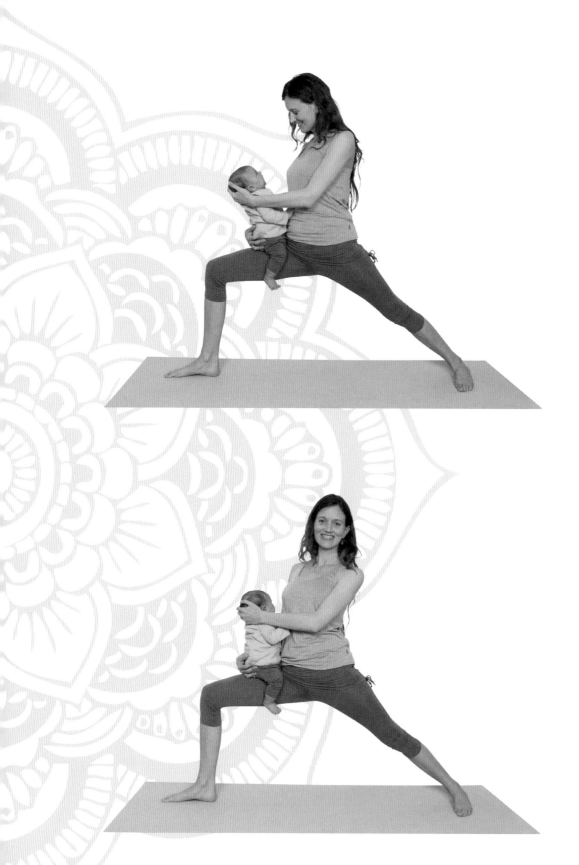

Virabhadrasana II with Baby

Warrior II Pose with Baby

In this adaptation you can hold your baby and simultaneously generate heat and strength.

Getting into the pose:

1. Stand in Tadasana in the middle of your sticky mat, holding baby.
2. Step into Utthita Hasta Padasana (p. 29).
3. Rotate into Parsva Hasta Padasana (p. 31).
4. Press firmly into the outer left foot and bend the right knee so that the center of the knee is in line with the center of the foot, and the knee is in line with the ankle.
5. Place baby on your right thigh, being sure to support his head if needed.
6. Keep the chest facing forward as much as possible.

Engaging actions

1. Draw the tailbone in and the sitting bones down.
2. Exhale; press the feet firmly down.
3. Inhale; lift and broaden the chest and firm the legs fully, especially the left thigh.
4. Keep the head in line with the spine and turn your head to look at your beautiful baby.
5. Soften your eyes, relax your face, and let the breath flow freely.

Stay for 5–10 breaths.

Coming out of the pose

Press your feet down and, keeping a strong hold of baby, straighten your right leg and step back to Tadasana.

Repeat on the other side.

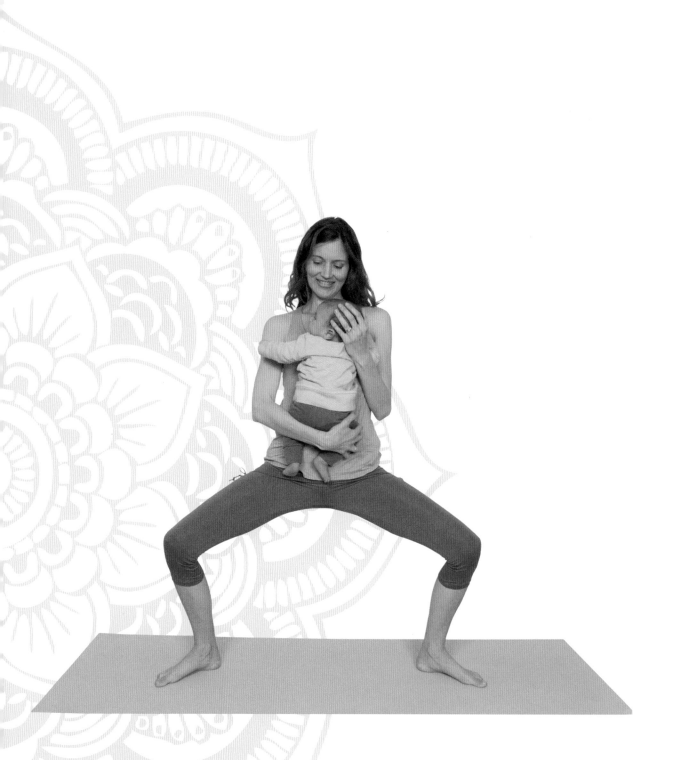

Half Squat

Half squats bring heat into your legs and also help to regain core strength. You can even bounce your baby at the same time—everyone is getting what they need! You can add this pose in at other times during your day when baby would like a bouncing motion, thereby bringing your yoga practice into your daily life.

Getting into the pose

1. Holding on to your baby securely, stand with your feet just wider than hip width apart and turn the toes out, away from your midline.
2. Bend your knees to come into a half squatting position.

Engaging actions

1. Draw the tailbone in and the sitting bones down.
2. Draw the heads of the shoulders back and down.
3. Exhale; press the heels firmly down.
4. Inhale; lift and broaden the chest.
5. Lift the pubic bone toward the navel.
6. If baby likes, you can bounce here.
7. Soften your eyes, relax your face, and let the breath flow freely.

Stay here for 5–10 breaths.

Coming out of the pose

Straighten the legs and rest a moment.

Repeat a few times.

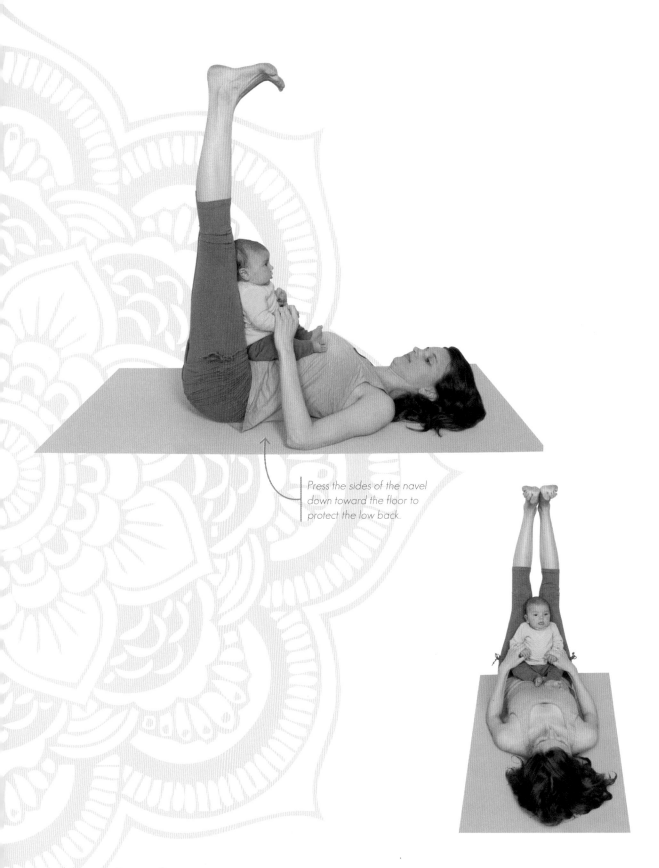

Press the sides of the navel down toward the floor to protect the low back.

Urdhva Prasarita Padasana with Baby

Upward Extended Foot Pose with Baby

This pose allows for lots of nice eye contact with baby while strengthening the abdominal muscles.

NOTE

It is important to wait at least 6–8 weeks after delivery before adding this pose into your practice; do not to practice this pose while there is postpartum bleeding. In cases of caesarean section, wait until the incision has fully healed before practicing this pose (at least 8 weeks).

GETTING INTO THE POSE

1. Lie down with your knees bent, feet on the floor, and place baby propped up against your thighs; keep holding on to baby throughout this pose.

2. Straighten your legs up to the ceiling so that your legs are perpendicular to the floor.

3. Keep your inner ankles together.

ENGAGING ACTIONS

1. Roll the thighs in to broaden the backs of the thighs and low back.

2. Press the sides of the navel down toward the floor.

3. Extend the legs fully; from the backs of the knees press firmly up through the heels. Press up through the big toe mounds.

Stay here for 10–15 breaths.

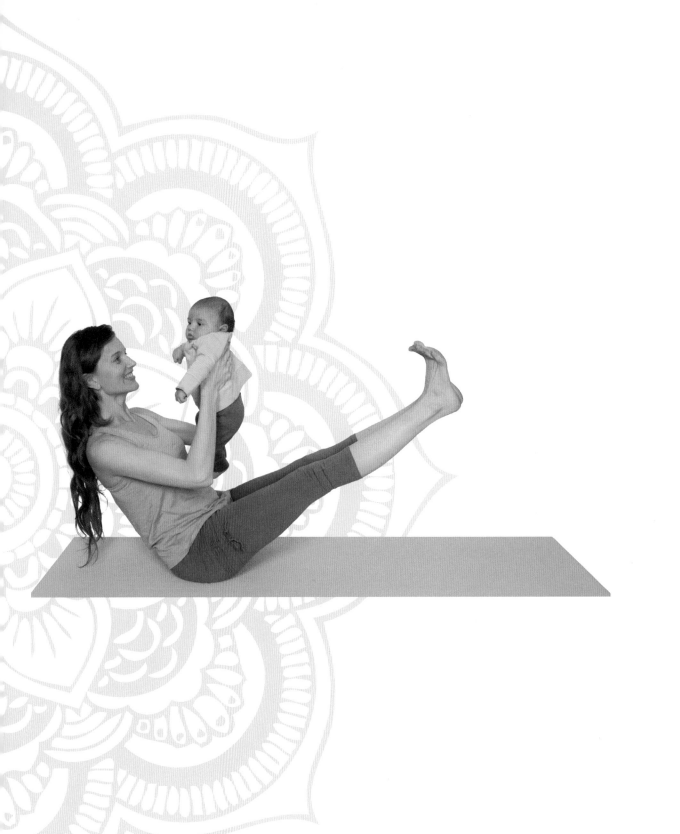

Paripurna Navasana with Baby

Boat Pose with Baby

In Paripurna Navasana, hang out with your baby and work your core at the same time! If you find straightening the legs too difficult, work on this pose with the knees bent.

NOTE

It is important to wait at least 6–8 weeks after delivery before adding this pose into your practice; do not to practice this pose while there is postpartum bleeding. In cases of caesarean section, wait until the incision has fully healed before practicing this pose (at least 8 weeks).

Also wait until baby has the strength to hold up his head on his own.

GETTING INTO THE POSE

1. Sit on the floor with your knees bent and baby sitting on your lap; hold onto baby's sides and chest area.
2. Holding on to baby, draw the shoulders back and down away from your ears to lift and broaden your chest.
3. Keep your chest open and lean back and balance on your sitting bones.
4. Straighten your legs fully.
5. Lift baby up so your arms are closely in line with the floor.

ENGAGING ACTIONS

1. Roll the front of the thighs in to broaden the backs of the legs.
2. Exhale; from the backs of your knees press out firmly through the inner heels and big toe mounds; press the sitting bones down evenly.
3. Inhale; lift and broaden the chest.
4. Firm your legs fully.

COMING OUT OF THE POSE

Bend your knees and place your feet back on the floor.

Try doing this pose multiple times.

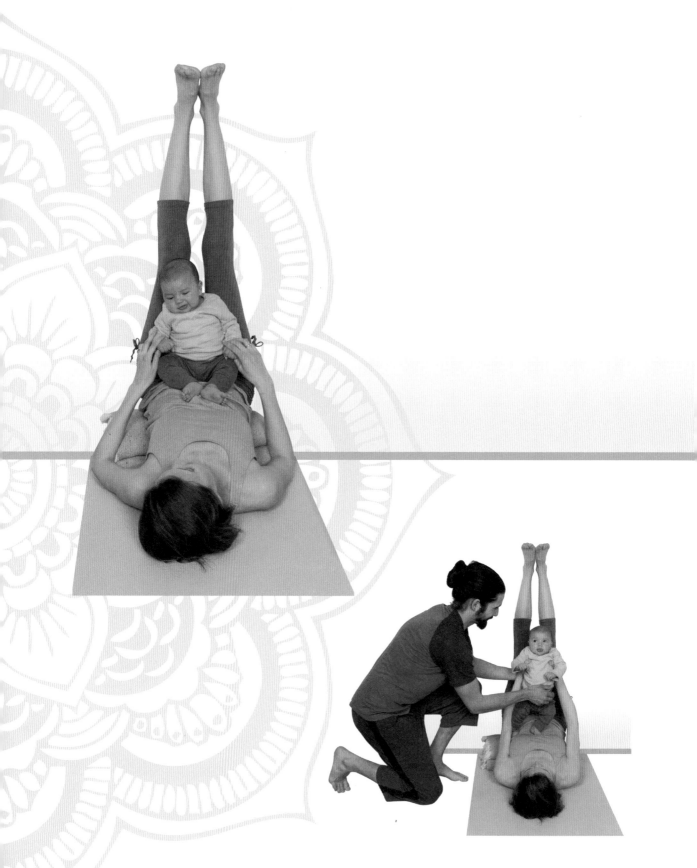

Viparita Karani with Baby
Inverted Seal Pose / Legs up the Wall Pose with Baby

When you are feeling exhausted and need to be refreshed, this is a fantastic aid. Babies often like sitting up like this too. You can also do this while baby is lying on your belly and nursing if it feels comfortable.

GETTING INTO THE POSE

1. Have baby on a blanket by your side so you can pick him up once you have gotten into the pose (unless someone is available to hand him to you).
2. Place two blankets in Basic Fold 4–6 inches away from the wall.
3. Sit on the blankets with your right hip against the wall.
4. Lie down on your left side and scoot your buttock to the wall.
5. Simultaneously swing your legs up against the wall and rotate your body so that both heels are on the wall and your back is on the floor.
6. Have the buttock just off the blankets toward the wall so there is a slight arch in the low back.
7. Pick up baby and place him sitting upright in your lap.

ENGAGING ACTIONS

1. Draw the shoulders away from the ears to open the chest; tuck the shoulder blades into the back to open the chest further.
2. Relax the inner groin down.

Stay for at least a few minutes and for as long as you and baby are happy.

COMING OUT OF THE POSE

Place baby back down on a blanket by your side; roll over to your side and pause for a moment before coming up to sitting.

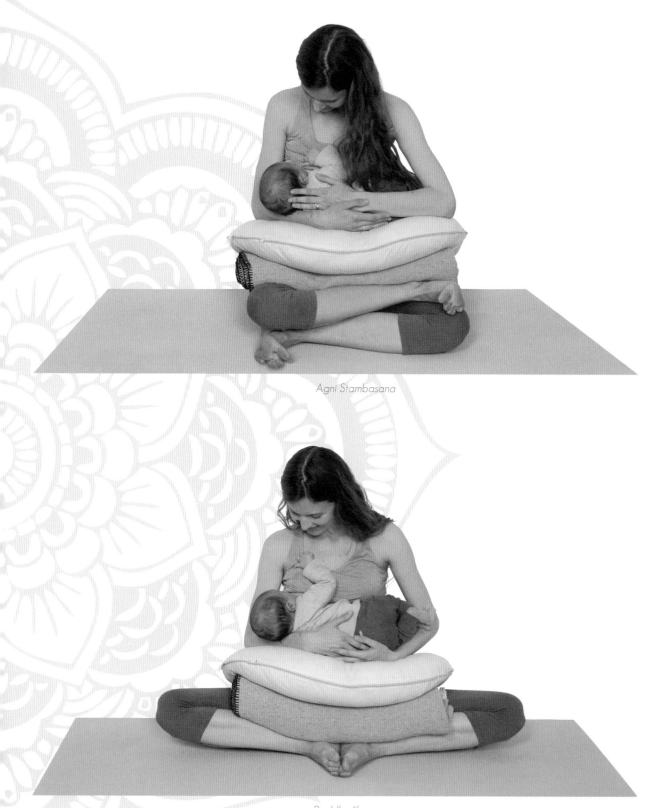

Agni Stambasana

Baddha Konasana

Breastfeeding Poses

Regardless of what physical position you are in, breastfeeding can be a yoga practice in and of itself. During the early days and months of adjusting to life with a new baby, the hours you spend nursing are perfect for quiet reflection and connection with yourself and your baby.

When you are ready, you can also get creative during breastfeeding and add in poses that open your hips or are restorative. In the first few months after baby is born it is best to avoid deep hip opening poses. The focus at this time is more on strengthening the legs and back, and doing gentle abdominal work when you are ready for it.

After a few months postpartum you can add in postures such as Agni Stambhasana (p. 101 and top left) or Baddha Konasana (p. 93 and bottom left), if you feel that your hips could use some release and opening. You could also try restoratives such as Supta Baddha Konasana (p. 135) or Viparita Karani (p. 147).

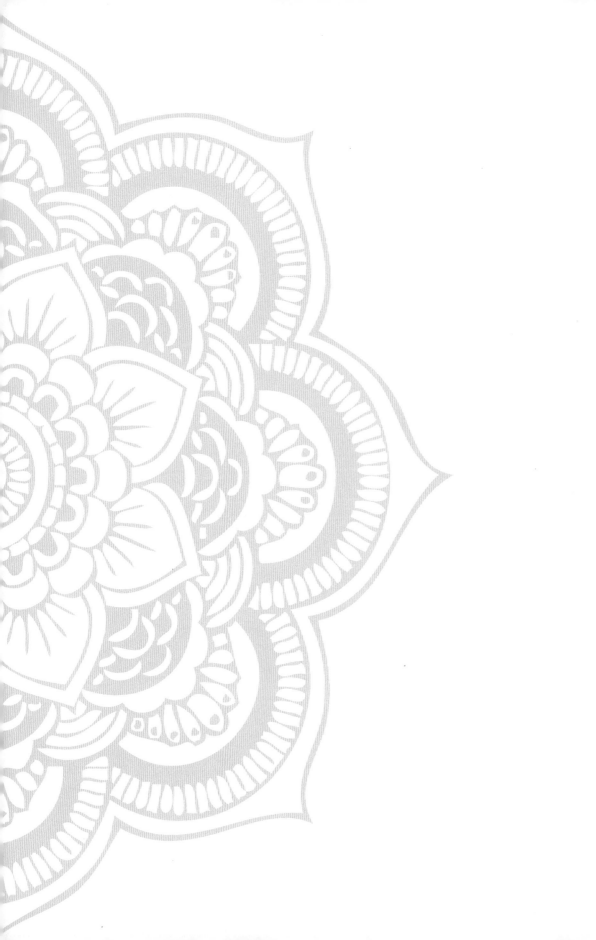

Postpartum Poses

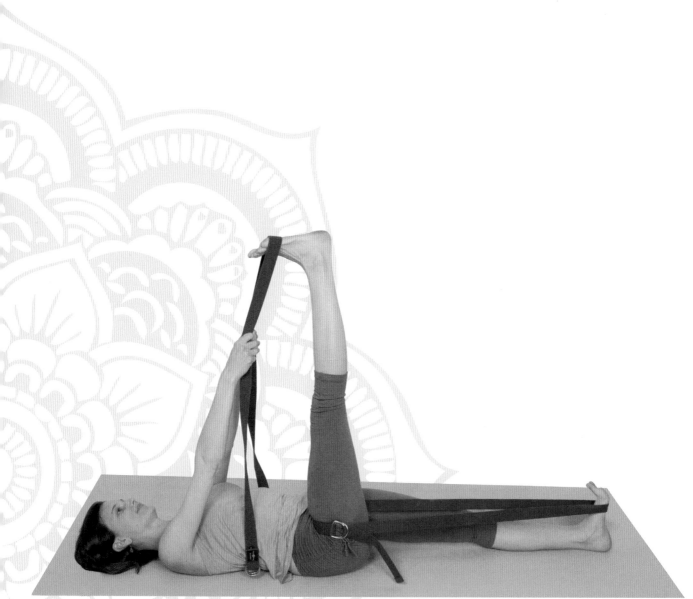

Supta Padangustasana Variation

Reclined Big Toe Foot Pose Variation

This variation of a Padangustasana uses two belts to stabilize the sacral area and is a great postpartum pose.

Getting into the pose

1. Make a large loop with one belt.
2. Lie down with your knees bent and feet flat on the floor.
3. Place the belt over the left big toe mound and the top of the right thigh all the way into the hip crease; have the buckle of the belt on the outside of the thigh with the tail of the belt pointing down toward your foot.
4. Straighten your left leg, being mindful that the left big toe is pointing straight up to the ceiling.
5. Tighten the belt by pulling the tail of the belt away from you, rotating your right thigh from inner to outer to take your right sit bone toward your feet.
6. Take the right knee in toward your chest; place a belt over the right big toe mound, holding onto the belt with both hands.
7. Straighten your right leg.
8. Walk your hands up the belt as close to the foot as possible.

Engaging actions

1. Rotate the upper arms away from one another and take the heads of the shoulders down to the floor and away from your ears to open and broaden the chest.
2. From the backs of the knees press strongly through the inner heels. Press out through the big toe mounds and firm the thighs.
3. Exhale; press the left inner thigh down to the floor; press the front of the right thigh to the back of the thigh to straighten the legs fully.
4. Inhale; keep opening and broadening the chest.
5. Soften your eyes, relax your face, and let the breath flow freely.

Stay in the pose for a minute or longer.

Coming out of the pose

Bend both knees, place the feet on the floor, and rest for a moment.

Repeat on the other side.

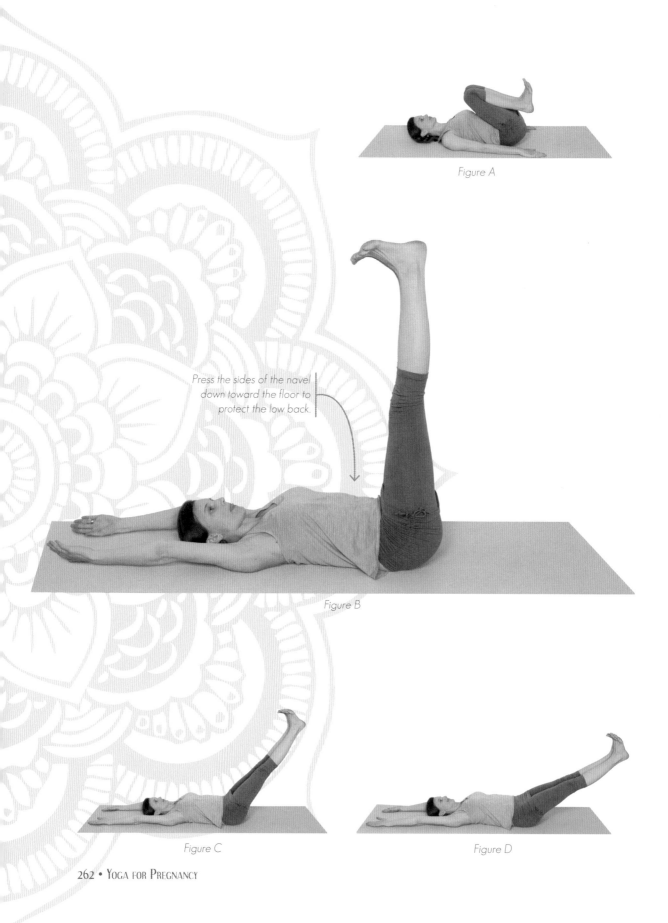

Figure A

Press the sides of the navel down toward the floor to protect the low back.

Figure B

Figure C

Figure D

Urdhva Prasarita Padasana
Upward Extended Foot Pose

This pose is strengthening to the abdominal muscles and generates heat and firmness in the core.

GETTING INTO THE POSE

1. Lie on the floor with your knees bent, feet on the floor, and arms by your sides.
2. Exhale; take the knees into the chest (*Figure A*).
3. Inhale; extend your arms up toward the ceiling and then down to the floor.
4. Turn your palms up to face the ceiling; have your wrists shoulder width apart (if the back of the hands do not reach the floor then place a blanket or two under your hands).
5. Straighten your legs up to the ceiling so that your legs are perpendicular to the floor; have your inner ankles together.

ENGAGING ACTIONS

1. Roll the thighs in to broaden the backs of the thighs and low back.
2. Press the sides of the navel down toward the floor.
3. Extend the legs fully; from the backs of the knees press firmly up through the heels. Press up through the big toe mounds and extend the arms and fingers all the way from the hips, lengthening the side body (*Figure B*).
4. Stay here for 10–15 breaths, then come down and rest for a few breaths.
5. Come into the pose again, legs at 90 degrees (perpendicular with the floor), following the above actions.
6. Keep the sides of the navel pressing to the floor and lower the legs to 60 degrees, or as far as you can without your lower back arching (*Figure C*).
7. Come down and rest.
8. Go into the pose again. If you can, bring the legs to 45 degrees, maintaining the action of the low back pressing to the floor (*Figure D*).
9. Rest lying flat on the floor for a few breaths.

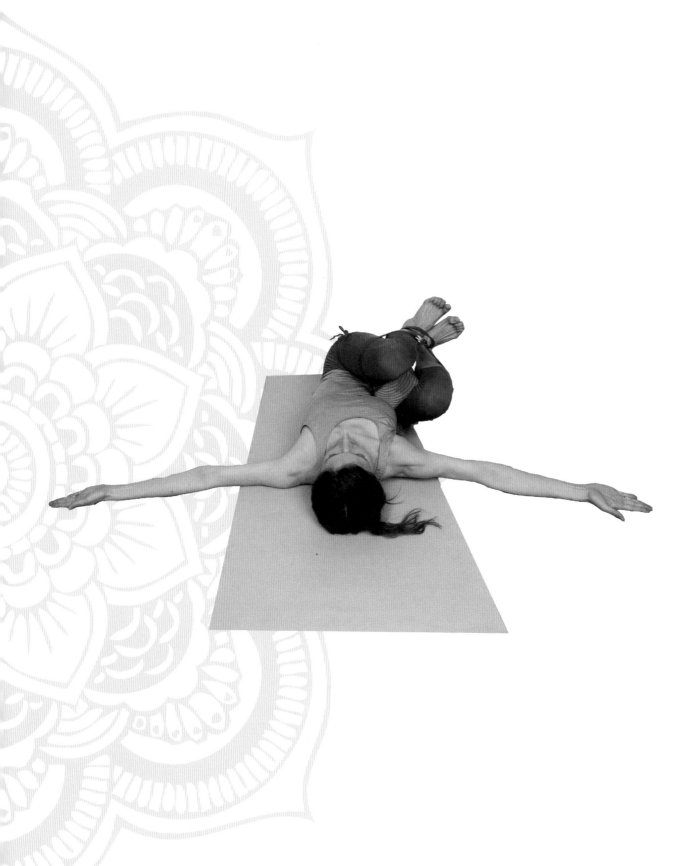

Jathara Parivartanasana
Stomach Rotating Pose

This pose strengthens the abdominal muscles, while the twisting action brings freedom to the spine.

NOTE

This pose can also be done without a block, but the block encourages inner thigh strength.

GETTING INTO THE POSE

1. Lie flat on the floor and bend your knees into your chest.
2. Place a block lengthwise between your thighs.
3. Stretch your arms out wide so the wrists are in line with your shoulders and the palms are facing the ceiling.
4. Press out through the big toe mounds and inner heels.

ENGAGING ACTIONS

1. Take a deep breath in, exhale, press the left shoulder and hand firmly down to the floor; take the knees up toward your right armpit and down toward the floor; do not take the legs all the way to the floor.
2. Press the thighs into the block.
3. From the outer left hip, extend through the outer left knee.
4. From the outer right knee, draw the leg back into the hip socket; be sure that the knees are in line with one another.
5. Press firmly out through the big toe mounds and inner heels.
6. Revolve the belly from right to left.
7. Soften your eyes, relax your face, and let the breath flow freely.

Stay for 3–4 breaths.

COMING OUT OF THE POSE

Take a deep breath in, then exhale and press the left hand strongly down and lead with the right thigh to come up to sitting.

Repeat on the other side.

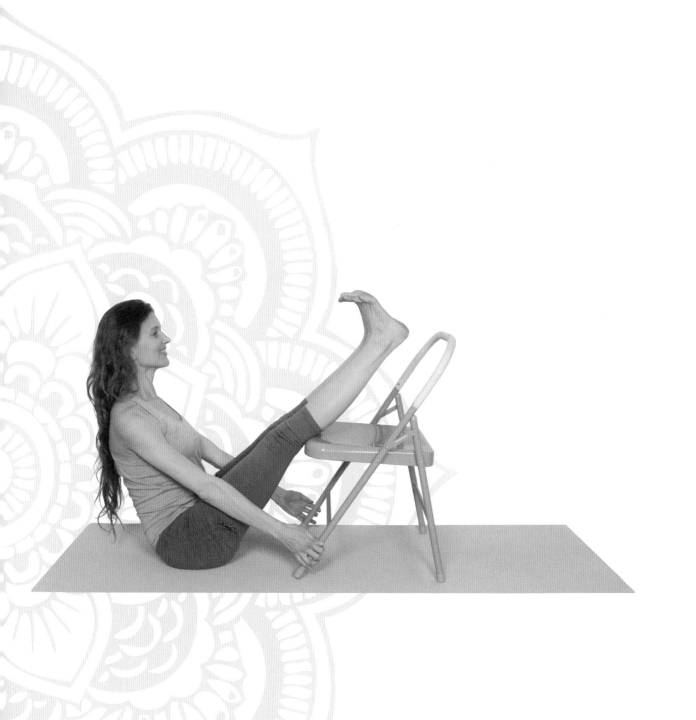

Paripurna Navasana Variation
Boat Pose Variation

This adaptation of boat pose is excellent for postpartum. It is a gentle way to begin adding some abdominal strengthening poses into your practice.

Getting into the Pose

1. Place a chair in the middle of your sticky mat with the seat facing toward you.
2. Place your calves on the seat of the chair and grip onto the front legs of the chair.

Engaging Actions

1. Roll your upper arms out, draw the shoulders down away from you ears, and lift and broaden the chest.
2. Straighten your legs; press out firmly through the inner heels and big toe mounds.
3. Lift the sternum bone higher.
4. Soften your eyes, relax your face, and let the breath flow freely.

Stay for 3–4 breaths.

Rest and repeat a few times.

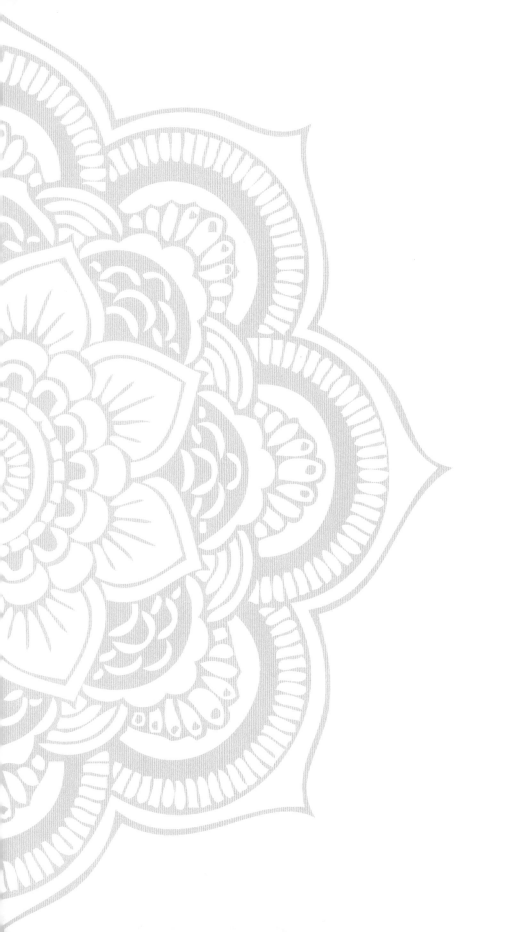

Partner Meditations

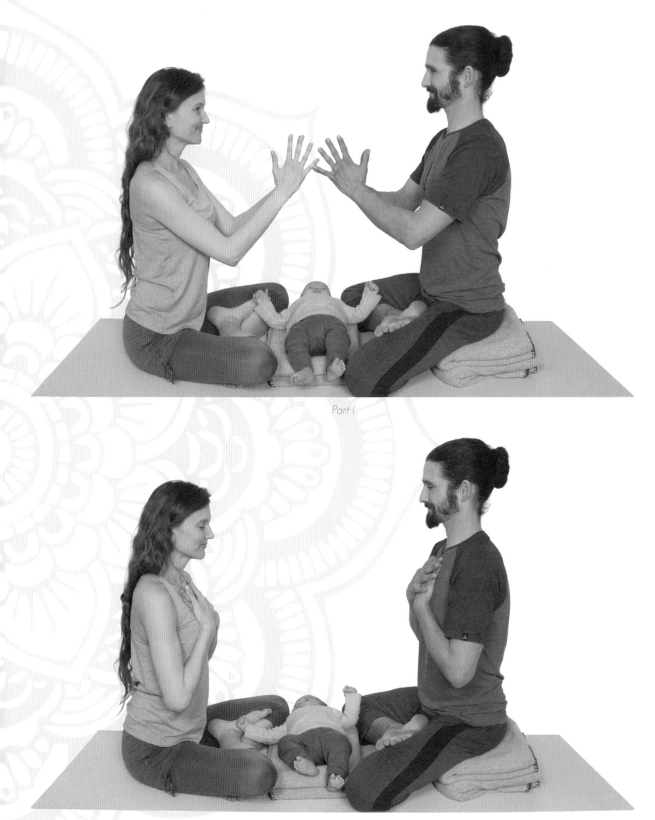

Part I

Part II

Shared Heart Meditation

Part I

Sit in a comfortable position facing each other. Have your knees about 8 inches apart. If you like, you can lay baby on a blanket in between you.

Press your palms together and spread the fingertips. Extend your arms out in front of you so that one of you has the middle outside edge of your pinky fingers resting on the other's pinky fingertips. Your elbows should be bent.

Draw your shoulders back and lift your chest. Soften your face, relax your throat, and let the breath flow freely. Gaze deeply into each other's eyes and radiate a sense of loving devotion toward one another. Stay here for a few minutes.

Part II

Close your eyes and bring your hands to cover your heart, left hand on the inside and right hand covering it. Spend a few minutes fully receiving the love and nurturing from your partner, and radiate some love into yourself as well.

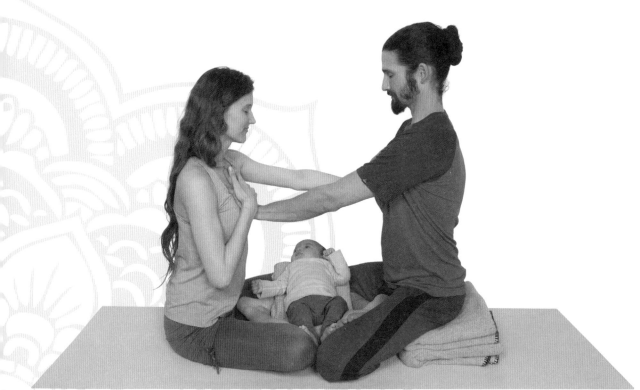

Part I

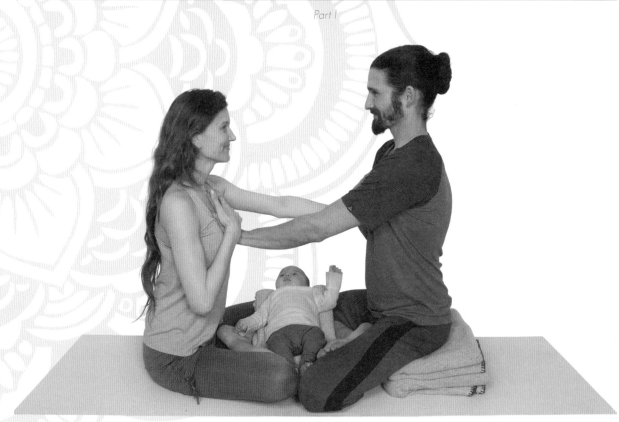

Part II

Circle of Support Meditation

PART I

Sit in a comfortable position facing each other. Have your knees touching. If you like, you can lay baby on a blanket in between you.

Place your right hand over your heart, and reach your left hand out to cover your partner's right hand.

Close your eyes. Soften your face, relax your throat, and let the breath flow freely. Feel the circle of energy flowing clockwise between you. Enjoy the feeling of support from your partner's hand over your heart. Stay here for a few minutes.

PART II

Open your eyes and let your gaze reflect support and love for your partner. A soft smile may come to your lips as you spend a few minutes experiencing the grace of quiet consciousness.

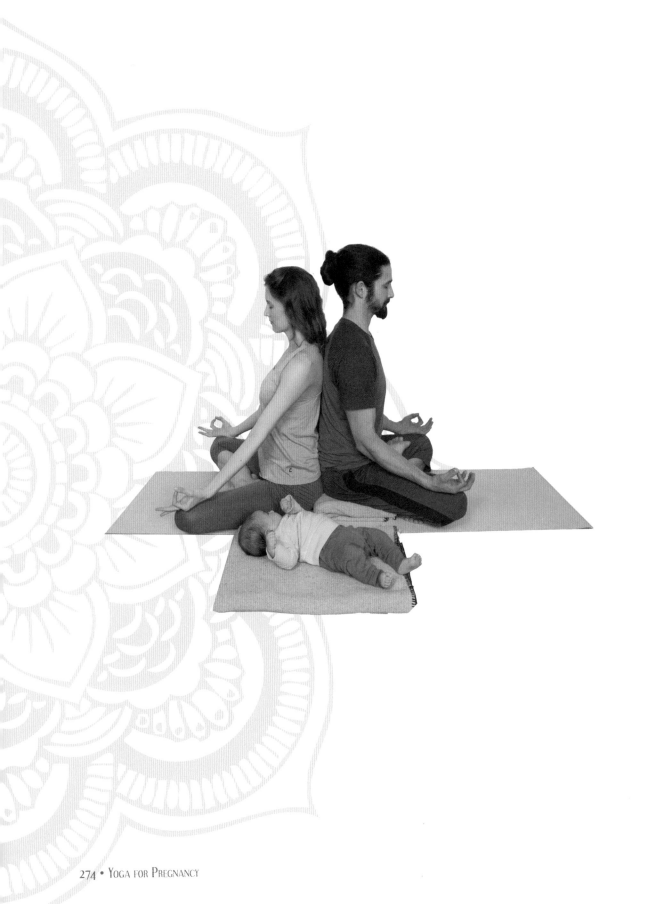

Unity Meditation

Sit in a comfortable position with your backs pressing together. If you like, you can lay baby on a blanket beside you.

Bring together the tip of the index finger and the tip of the thumb. Relax your other fingers and let the backs of your hands rest on your knees.

Close your eyes and drop your chin slightly. Keeping the chin tucked, draw your shoulders back and lift your chest. Soften your face, relax your throat, and let the breath flow freely. Rest in the support of your spine aligned with your partner's. Stay here for a few minutes.

Acknowledgments

From Leslie

It is with deep heartfelt gratitude that I would like to give thanks to my teacher Ingela Abbott. I am continually inspired by your overflowing love and wisdom of the Iyengar yoga method and your strong dedicated practice of over forty years. It is a rare gift to find a teacher like you and I feel very fortunate to have found you.

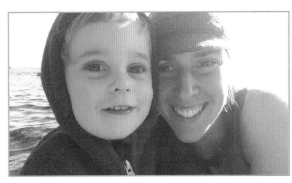

Salish and Leslie

I am profoundly grateful to the life long work of Guruji BKS Iyengar for the gift of yoga to the world. It is of great honor that I have the privelege to continue on this practice you have so skillfully mastered and taught. May we all practice in the dedication for a more peaceful, whole, and happy inner and outer world.

I would like to give a big thanks to my incredibly supportive husband, Orion. Thank you for unquestionable unconditional love. Thank you for always doing what it takes to make my dreams come true. You are a gem of a man, Orion. You are a beautiful father. I am so blessed to be your wife. I love you.

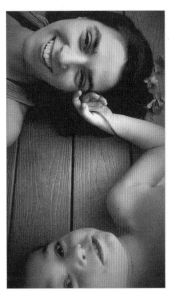

Leslie and Kosta

Thank you to my two beautiful little boys, Kosta and Salish. I look at your sweet little faces every day and it reminds me of how amazing and precious life really is. You are my wise teachers. I thank my lucky stars every day for having you both in my life.

Thank you, Joan and Craig Williams, for being great examples of loving parents and now grandparents. I love you two more than words can express.

Jill, I cherish our sisterhood. Thanks for always teaching me to smile and for your support through this whole process. I love you!

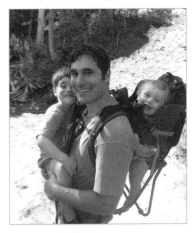

Kosta, Orion, and Salish

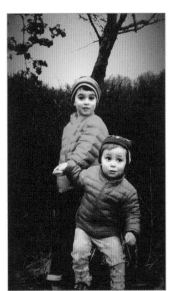

Kosta and Salish

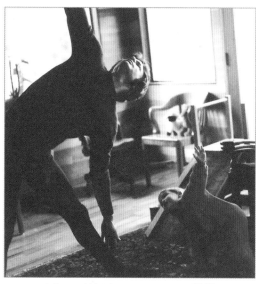

John and Noah practicing yoga, 1982

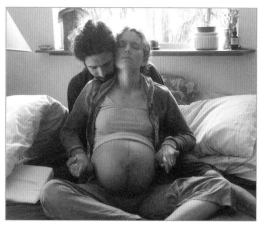

Noah providing support during labor

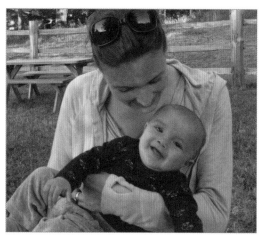

Robin Wilder Westgate at 4½ months

From Megan

I am so grateful to my son's grandparents for exposing both his father and me to meditation and yoga from a young age. One of my earliest memories is of "Om-ing" with my sister and mother at bedtime, and I grew up being taught to respect and care for myself, mind, body, and spirit. My husband was also raised with these values, as can be seen from this photo of him at age 2 practicing triangle pose with his papa. This picture has special significance because of the heartbreaking fact that we lost Noah's father, John Westgate, during the writing of this book, just eleven days before our first son was born. He was a tender, peaceful soul whose example we continue to learn from every day.

To my beloved husband and divine playmate, Noah: Thank you from the bottom of my heart for all of the ways you inspire me to live my yoga. Human embodiment (and parenthood!) is certainly not without its challenges, but there is no one I would rather learn these lessons with than you. There is also no one I would rather make babies with, and what an amazing start we are off to!

Robin Wilder Westgate, your sparkling spirit takes my breath away. I am humbled in the face of your radiance and am so profoundly grateful to look forward to a life of learning and growing with you. I love you more than words can say.

Thank you also to the personal teachers, scholars, and great yogis who have inspired me and given me a path to follow, especially Krishna Das, B.K.S. Iyengar, Stephen Cope, Pema Chödrön, Ingela Abbott, Georg Feuerstein, Scott Traffas, MC Yogi & Amanda, Carey Wright, Danielle LaPorte, Gurmukh, Gayna Uransky, Janice Steinem, Chip Hartranft, Eckhart Tolle, and Patanjali. Jai!

RESOURCES AND REFERENCES

Cope, Stephen. *The Wisdom of Yoga: A Seeker's Guide to Extraordinary Living*. New York: Bantam Books, 2006.

Das, Krishna. *The Flow of Grace: Chanting the Hanuman Chalisa, Entering into the Presence of the Powerful, Compassionate Being Known as Hanuman*. Boulder, CO: Sounds True, 2007.

Feuerstein, Georg. *The Path of Yoga: An Essential Guide to Its Principles and Practices*. Boston: Shambhala, 2011.

Feuerstein, Georg. *The Shambhala Encyclopedia of Yoga*. Boston: Shambhala, 2000.

Gaskin, Ina May. *Ina May's Guide to Childbirth*. New York: Bantam Books, 2003.

Iyengar, B. K. S. *Light on Pranayama: The Yogic Art of Breathing*. New York: Crossroad, 2002.

Iyengar, B. K. S. *Light on Yoga: Yoga Dipika*. New York: Schocken Books, 1979.

Iyengar, Geeta S., Rita Keller, and Kerstin Khattab. *Iyengar Yoga for Motherhood: Safe Practice for Expectant & New Mothers*. New York: Sterling, 2010.

Iyengar, Geeta S. *Yoga, a Gem for Women*. New Delhi: Allied Publishers Private, 1983.

Judith, Anodea. *Wheels of Life: A User's Guide to the Chakra System*. St. Paul, MN: Llewellyn Publications, 1987.

Khalsa, Gurmukh Kaur. *Bountiful, Beautiful, Blissful: Experience the Natural Power of Pregnancy and Birth with Kundalini Yoga*. New York: Griffin, 2004.

Khalsa, Shakta Kaur. *Kundalini Yoga as Taught by Yogi Bhajan: Unlock Your Inner Potential through Life-changing Exercise*. New York: Dorling Kindersley Publications, 2001.

Patañjali, and Chip Hartranft. *The Yoga-Sutra of Patañjali: A New Translation with Commentary*. Boston, MA: Shambhala Publications, 2003.

Yoga in Action: Intermediate Course-1 by Geeta S. Iyengar.

Yoga in Action: Preliminary Course by Geeta S. Iyengar.

Index